PHYSICAL ACTIVITIES IN THE WHEELCHAIR AND OUT

An Illustrated Guide to Personalizing Participation

E. Ann Davis, MS

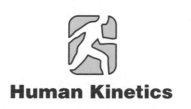

Human Kinetics

Library of Congress Cataloging-in-Publication Data

Davis, E. Ann, 1949-
   Physical activities in the wheelchair and out : an illustrated guide to personalizing participation / E. Ann Davis.
      p. cm.
   ISBN-13: 978-1-4504-0199-9 (soft cover)
   ISBN-10: 1-4504-0199-6 (soft cover)
   1. Students with disabilities--Education--United States--Handbooks, manuals, etc. 2. Students with disabilities--Orientation and mobility--United States--Handbooks, manuals, etc. 3. Teaching--Aids and devices--United States--Handbooks, manuals, etc. 4. Activity programs in education--United States--Handbooks, manuals, etc. 5. Wheelchairs I. Title.
   LC4031.D38 2011
   371.90973--dc23

                              2011017939

ISBN-10: 1-4504-0199-6 (print)
ISBN-13: 978-1-4504-0199-9 (print)

Copyright © 2012 by E. Ann Davis

The anecdotes in this book are all true, but the names are fictional.

Acquisitions Editor: Cheri Scott; **Developmental Editor:** Jacqueline Eaton Blakley; **Assistant Editor:** Anne Rumery; **Copyeditor:** Mary Rivers; **Illustrator:** © E. Ann Davis; **Graphic Designer:** Joe Buck; **Graphic Artist:** Yvonne Griffith; **Cover Designer:** Keith Blomberg; **Art Manager:** Kelly Hendren; **Associate Art Manager:** Alan L. Wilborn; **Printer:** United Graphics

Printed in the United States of America

10 9 8 7 6 5 4 3 2 1

The paper in this book is certified under a sustainable forestry program.

Human Kinetics
Web site: www.HumanKinetics.com

United States: Human Kinetics
P.O. Box 5076
Champaign, IL 61825-5076
800-747-4457
e-mail: humank@hkusa.com

Canada: Human Kinetics
475 Devonshire Road Unit 100
Windsor, ON N8Y 2L5
800-465-7301 (in Canada only)
e-mail: info@hkcanada.com

Europe: Human Kinetics
107 Bradford Road
Stanningley
Leeds LS28 6AT, United Kingdom
+44 (0) 113 255 5665
e-mail: hk@hkeurope.com

Australia: Human Kinetics
57A Price Avenue
Lower Mitcham, South Australia 5062
08 8372 0999
e-mail: info@hkaustralia.com

New Zealand: Human Kinetics
P.O. Box 80
Torrens Park, South Australia 5062
0800 222 062
e-mail: info@hknewzealand.com

E5300

Contents

Foreword

Lauren J. Lieberman, PhD

I have taught children with severe and multiple disabilities for many years in inclusive and segregated settings. Thinking of ways to involve children with physical disabilities in activities in any placement of physical education has been a struggle for teachers for years.

Ann Davis has written a book to embrace, excite, and challenge teachers as they include children with physical disabilities in physical education. The creativity, imagination, and commitment that Ann shows through *Physical Activities In the Wheelchair and Out* are incredible. You can see the results of her years of teaching and success throughout this book.

Ann is an alumna of the College at Brockport, where I teach, and she has taught children with physical disabilities for many years. When she was looking for an outlet for a book she had developed from her years of teaching children with special needs, she sent me a draft. I immediately said that she had to get these ideas out to teachers. The ideas are clear, practical, and applicable to children of any age. Teachers have been longing for a book like this for years.

This book is unique: It focuses on children with severe and multiple disabilities who may or may not use wheelchairs. The upbeat graphics clearly explain how to set up an activity or game. Each skill or game is presented in several ways to accommodate the variety of abilities we see daily in our gymnasiums. The participants can choose whether to use their chairs, depending on their goals. The graphics in the book are so good that they can be used in stations to show the skill or activity to be performed, and they are so clear that a volunteer, paraeducator, or trained peer tutor could use them as a guide to activity stations with one child or a group of children.

Another unique aspect of this book is that it offers activities for individual, partner, or group configurations. These include activities for body awareness, body control, manipulative activities, and games. *Physical Activities In the Wheelchair and Out* focuses on personalizing participation using the variables of space, equipment, and skill performance. Each activity, whether it is a push, drop, throw, catch, or strike, shows skills from simple to complex, using common equipment that you most likely have in your program.

The games section of the book describes simple games that teachers can offer in their segregated or inclusive classes. Games like beanbag race, punch volleyball, hit and run, gone fishing, knock-down relay race, ball dance, and many more are explained with both in-the-chair and out-of-the-chair versions. They focus on basic game, sport, and recreation skills that will help children throughout their lives.

Whether you are a teacher, parent, teacher aid, therapist, or professional preparation student, *Physical Activities In the Wheelchair and Out* will open up your mind and excite your imagination. With a little time, energy, and innovation, all of your students will be active participants in any game or activity that is in your curriculum!

I would like to thank Ann personally for her dedication and commitment to the field. Her creativity, energy, enthusiasm, and passion can now be shared with others through this amazing book of games and activities, *in the wheelchair and out*!

Preface

Most of us move our bodies and their parts with little or no attention to the fact that our effortless movement is a gift. Thus, it's easy for us to take for granted all the benefits that physical activity adds to our lives. However, there are those for whom even minor movements require major effort. They, too, deserve the benefits of physical activity, activities that are constructed to use their abilities as they are.

In this book, you will find ideas that provide opportunities for individuals with disabilities to develop basic participation skills in ways that meet their unique abilities. Full of physical activities and games that can be done in a wheelchair (or any chair) and on the floor, it has been written with the emphasis on adapting activity to participants' differing performance abilities. This book minimizes performance guidelines, benchmarks, and outcomes that usually require individuals to conform to a standard. Instead, it describes activities that participants can perform in ways that are most suitable for them.

This book will help teachers, therapists, caregivers, recreation specialists, and others develop modified and adapted activities. It offers alternatives and techniques that promote independent participation and presents them in enjoyable and creative ways. The activities described allow unique participation methods that emphasize abilities rather than disabilities, strengths versus weaknesses, leading to good feelings about movement. There is joy in physical activity, and we, as teachers and caregivers, are responsible for finding ways for those with limitations to share that joy.

The design of this book keeps words to a minimum; instead, it uses illustrations to show many ways to present skills and games. Because each day brings new opportunities and challenges, activities need continued revision if they are to be successful when we are working with those with disabilities. The illustrations provided in this book are meant to be a springboard for your own creative thought as you work each day with students of varying and changing needs.

The activities presented here are suitable for those with limited physical skills and delayed or poor motor coordination and control, as well as those who have normal developmental skills. The activities can provide the impetus for participation in adaptive physical education, therapeutic recreation, home play, and all areas where physical activity is encouraged. The activities are doable, allowing those with developmental disabilities as well as those disabled through life circumstances to experience physical success.

An individual does not have to be in a wheelchair to benefit from the activities described here; individuals who do not normally use a wheelchair can also benefit from doing activities in a seated position. A chair can provide personal boundaries for an individual. A chair can remove interfering issues such as poor balance. A chair can level the playing field in multilevel groups. A chair can limit other distractions. A chair can assist an individual in organizing the immediate environment.

Providing activities that allow for success on personal terms encourages a positive attitude about one's individual capabilities. Besides the obvious physical benefit of participation is the additional one of feeling good about oneself, enjoying a sense of accomplishment, and having fun.

This book will help you develop active participants who are comfortable with who they are and confident in spite of limitations. Movement is the heart of physical education and recreation and plays a major role in health. Positive self-image and self-confidence are also components of good health. Humans come in a variety of sizes, shapes, and abilities. As a person working with individuals with disabilities, you have a unique opportunity to develop participation styles that encourage success by recognizing differences that honor the amazing diversity of human beings.

Acknowledgments

Thank you to Dr. Judy Jensen, Sonia Sumar, The Prospect Child and Family Center, and Dr. Lauren Lieberman. Each came into my life at a different time, and every time was just the right time.

A special thanks to the teaching assistants and teachers who supported and enhanced my years in adapted physical education. You made it possible for so many children to experience success.

Thank you to all the children who let me work with the body to connect with the soul.

Using This Guide

Physical Activities In the Wheelchair and Out: An Illustrated Guide to Personalizing Participation shows you a general approach to adaptive activity that you can use with any participant in any context. The principle of using the same organization, rules, and methodology to keep things fair and even is actually unfair to many participants. Acknowledging differences and honoring uniqueness by providing opportunities to participate in one's own way respects the dignity of those with disabilities. In any given activity, several participants may access and perform the activity in several different ways. The idea of customizing each activity for each participant might seem overwhelming at first, but this book will spark your own creativity with ideas and variations and provide a foundation of knowledge that you can build on as you gain experience.

PROGRESSION

Because body awareness is a prerequisite for other physical skills and activities, chapter 1 is devoted to exploring concepts and vocabulary related to body parts, movement, and spatial awareness. Subsequent chapters explore various manipulative skills (such as kicking and throwing) in the same way, defining the skill and illustrating ways in which the skill can be practiced in the chair or on the floor. The final chapter brings body awareness and skills together in group games.

The book is based on the premise that individual skill precedes the organization and interaction necessary for partner and group activity. Body awareness, actions, and control are the basics needed for more complex activities. Individual success in these areas leads to the ability to participate with another person. This then leads to group activities, games, and modified sports that require not only basic skills but interaction with others and a higher level of organization.

Each chapter shows individual activities first and then activities that can be done with partners. Each chapter begins by breaking a skill into its simplest components and then offering progressive alternatives in the execution of the skill. Hints for implementation are also included. Following the description of the skill and its options are the actual activity ideas. The illustrations are meant to offer suggestions and, for the most part, do not reflect individual modifications and adaptations. Performance of the activity will need to be individualized using the suggested options as well as the current abilities of each participant.

The organization used in this book follows a logical progression. Using the skill of kick as an example, the curricular progression would be as follows:

1. Activities that teach and encourage the use of the feet and legs conducted in centers or any loose formation that has individual participation as its focus
2. The addition of a ball, beanbag, or other object that can be moved with the legs or feet during the activity, still requiring solitary engagement
3. Simple partner activities using the legs or feet that include a ball or beanbag and cooperative play

4. Simple group games played in a line, circle, or scatter formation that, in part or as a whole, use a ball, beanbag, or object moved with the legs or feet

5. Lead-up games and modified sports that primarily use the legs and feet

Participants in this series of activities are provided with a progressive experience in skill, social interaction, and complexity of organization as each step adds a layer of difficulty. Partner play requires individual skill and a certain social awareness. Group games add additional requirements such as waiting for a turn or staying in a specific formation. Lead-up games and modified sports call for specific roles, actions and patterns, rules, and often the performance of two or more differing actions in the same activity.

PERSONALIZATION

Personalizing participation involves using the tools of space, equipment, and skill in unique ways that meet the abilities of each person. Each of these tools plays a vital role in success, and none are an end in themselves. They are all a means to an end and provide the key to successful participation.

Space

Space requirements in an activity depend on range of motion, ability to impart force, speed of movement, and ability to understand boundaries. Here are some general guidelines for using space to adapt activities:

- Clearly mark activity areas to define boundaries and participation requirements within the space.
- Evaluate the spatial needs of each person. Some participants may need to be closer to activity components. Some may need to travel shorter distances. Some may need items to be higher or placed closer to the ground.
- Decrease the overall activity space when necessary to facilitate successful participation. Use a smaller court, a lower net, a smaller circle, or closer bases.
- During initial trials of an activity, err on the side of less space rather than more. Distances can be modified for the group and per individual as needed.
- Placement of the chair in relation to the activity affects the ability to perform.
  - Adjust the angle of the chair and its proximity to equipment and supports for each person.
  - Some activities may work better with the wheelchair in an upright position, others with the chair tilted back.
  - Chairs may need to be turned sideways to facilitate use of a dominant side of the body.
  - In some types of activities, chairs may need to be touching to encourage successful participation.
  - Position chairs nearer to or farther from light sources, sounds, other participants, and equipment to accommodate individual needs.

Equipment

It's important to select the right equipment for each person. Like clothing, equipment can be too big, too small, too heavy, or too light for the conditions. Whether participants will be able to use equipment that is of standard size and weight will depend on the disability. Equipment is a means to an end. Adapt and substitute in order to reach those ends.

Within the range of standard equipment items, there are many potential adjustments that can be made:

- An activity that uses a ball can use a basketball, volleyball, playground ball, semi-inflated ball, slow-moving ball, oversized ball, heavy ball, light ball, or even a balloon.
  - Hanging a ball eliminates the need to chase and retrieve. Hang balls from the ceiling, basketball hoops, or chin-up bars.
  - For two-hand throws, use a ball that can be slightly compressed to help with grip.
  - Punchballs (purchased in the party supply area of stores) or balloons are slower moving, lighter, and easier to track, and they move easily with minimal force applied. They are a good option when range of motion is an issue.
  - Less air in a ball makes for better grip, less bounce, and a shorter distance traveled.
- In activities that use an implement for striking, any of the following will work: a paddle, a bat, a dowel rod, a paper towel tube, a rhythm stick, one's own hand, one's hand with a puppet on it, or a plastic bowling pin.
  - A thin bat or dowel rod can be easier to grasp.
  - A fat bat and a large ball give the greatest potential contact area.
  - A paddle or short bat is easier to move in the desired direction.
  - A racket provides a large surface area for striking.
  - Support equipment for striking, such as batting tees and balls suspended by rope or string, should be placed in the way that best works for each person. Distance, height, and placement in relation to the chair need to be considered. Some participants will be more successful with supports placed in front of them and some with the supports placed to the side. Experiment to see what works best.

Equipment choices are a part of the process of individualizing participation. The same equipment does not have to be used for each player even though the activity or game is the same for all.

Skill

The importance of developing methods that increase independent participation in physical activities cannot be stressed enough. In instances where there is limited mobility, it becomes imperative to structure techniques to meet the immediate capabilities of the participant. To learn by doing is to experience and organize firsthand single or sequential movements. Skill is acquired in many ways. Find these ways, often through trial and error, and assist the participant in building a repertoire of activities that can be done individually or with others. As competence is established, technique can become more focused and refined. Additional time, many repetitions, and assistance, provided as needed, lead to greater participation ability. Begin with what is and work toward what could be. Performance skill is another tool, a means to an end. And the end is always to cultivate the most independent participation possible for each person.

Consider the following general guidelines for modifying skill execution:

- Assess what movement is possible, right down to eye blinks, head nods, and smiles.

- Demonstrate first, and then offer physical assistance.

- Physical assistance is a means to an end, a learning tool. It is not a participation method. Every time there is physical assistance, there should be give and take between the participant and the person providing the assistance. In cases of severe disability, having the opportunity to indicate readiness for play by facial expression, eye contact, or sound may be the only independent participation possible.

- Break the action into simple steps and verbalize *what* body parts are moving as well as *how* they are moving.

- Simplify skills by providing cue words for each major step in the action. For example, for the overhand throw, say, "Up. Throw." Use the fewest words that make sense to cue the action.

- Position the wheelchair to facilitate performance of the skill.

- In body awareness activities, looking at, pointing to, or moving a part are all acceptable ways of indicating awareness.

- Performance of a skill after a period of practice compared to the initial performance of the skill may show only small, if any, variation. Over time the ability to perform an action will improve, but the performance of a skill will always be individual.

- Gradations in movement components such as speed, force, and direction before and after practice may be minimal. Investigate these components individually, finding the best way for a participant to impart force, increase speed, or control direction (overhand, underhand, sidearm, and so on).

- When demonstrating an action, use a lot of space. Exaggerated movements are more visible and show smaller components more easily. Move slowly when demonstrating.

Use combinations of space, equipment, and skill execution that work for the individual participant. Finding ways for each person to experience success requires patience. It also entails letting go of standard rules for skill execution and, instead, being creative. Look at the function of the skill first. How can a person meet the function of the skill when the execution of the standard form is not within current abilities? To paraphrase William James, "If it works, it's true."

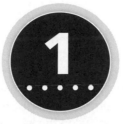

BODY AWARENESS

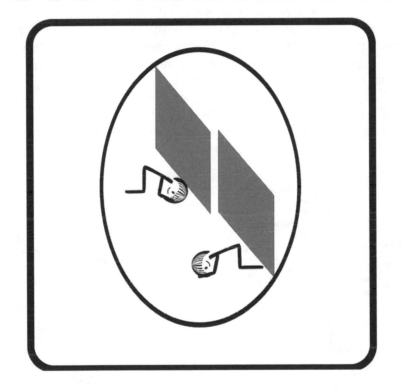

I once demonstrated how to do a headstand against the wall in a class of mobile students with special needs. When asked to try it, one participant placed his head and hands against the wall, waited, then turned around and placed his feet against the wall. He then turned again and went back to his original position. He stayed there for a moment and then reversed again, placing his feet to the wall. He understood that both the head and feet ended up at the wall, but he had no concept of how to get his body in that position.

It is important to remember that when mobility is limited, exploration of the environment is also limited. Normal development of body awareness can be compromised by the inability to explore one's self and environment. Kinesthetic awareness (awareness of the position of the body in space) can also be compromised.

It is important to spend time reinforcing basic body awareness as well as spatial awareness. Provide activities that develop the awareness of body parts, movement of parts, and movement of the whole body. Terms like *front* and *back*, *up* and *down*, *top* and *bottom*, *next to*, *in front of*, *in back of*, *side*, *near*, *far*, *over*, *under*, *forward*, *backward*, and *sideways* are all concepts that need to be reinforced, if not taught directly.

Without these simple concepts, it is difficult to follow directions for movement. When we teach a skill, we use spatial terms. But if the participant does not understand the term *backward*, saying, "Move your leg backward to prepare to kick," is ineffective. Thus, it is important to spend time teaching and reviewing on a regular basis the most common terms.

Teach body awareness through individual and partner activities and employ the use of basic and easily manageable equipment to keep experiences fresh. Encourage the use of as many body parts as possible when performing whole-body movements such as wiggle or shake.

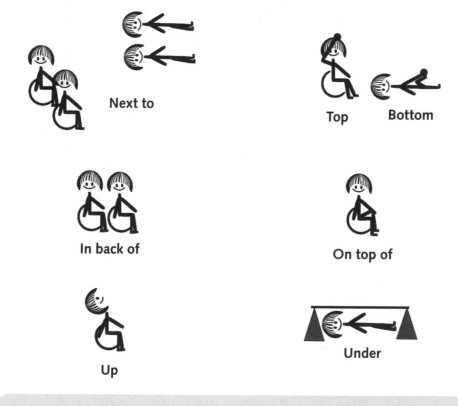

Next to

Top   Bottom

In back of

On top of

Up

Under

Teaching movement provides us with the opportunity to see the thinking process as it happens.

BODY PARTS

Head

Elbow

Knee

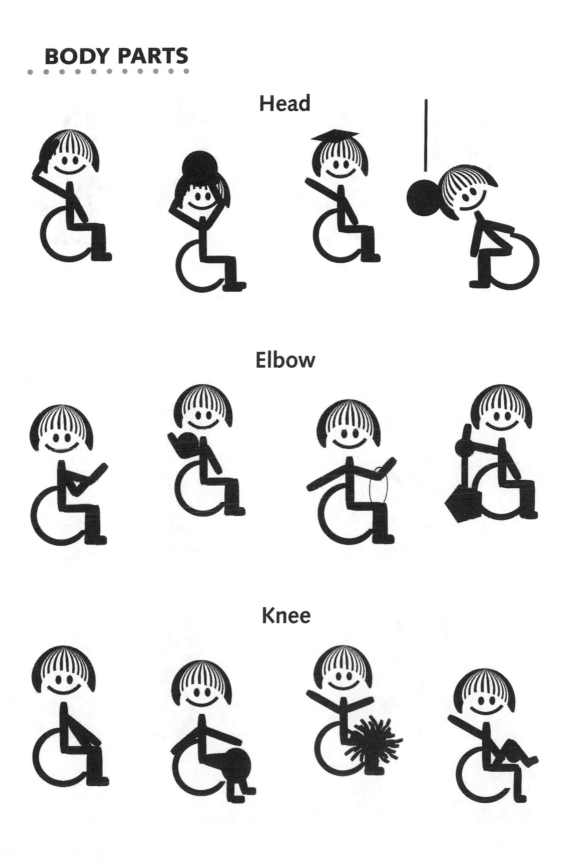

Foot

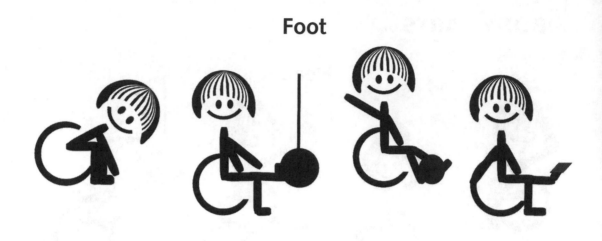

PARTS WITH PARTS

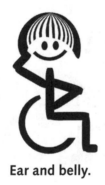

Ear and belly.

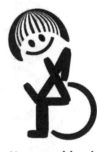

Knee and back.

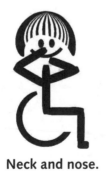

Neck and nose.

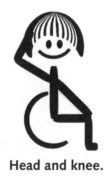

Head and knee.

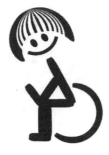

Elbows to knees.

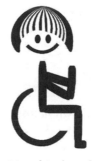

Hand to hand.

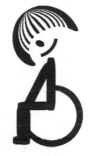

Chin to chest.

Leg to knee.

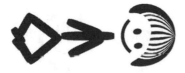

Foot to foot.

Hand to ankle.

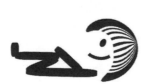

Knees to chest.

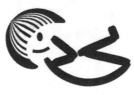

Elbow to knee.

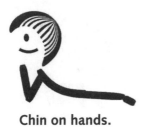

Chin on hands.

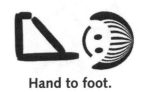

Hand to foot.

PARTNER PARTS

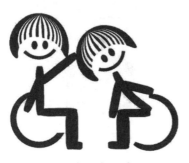

Hand to head.

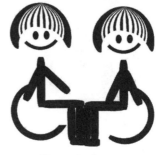

Knee to knee.

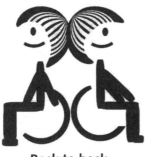

Back to back.

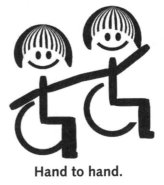

Hand to hand.

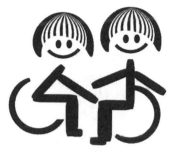

Hand to knee.

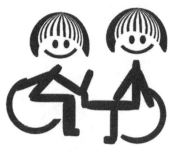

Elbow to foot.

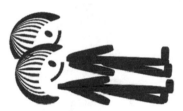

Side to side.

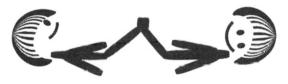

Foot to foot.

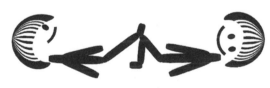

Foot to knee.

Hand to hand.

INDIVIDUAL BODY ACTIONS

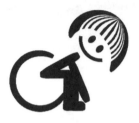

Bend.

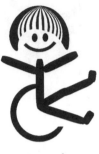

Stretch.

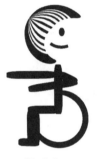

Twist.

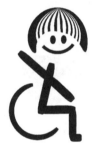

Rock.

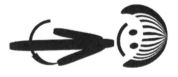

Roll.

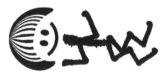

Shake.

Kick.

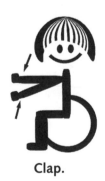

Clap.

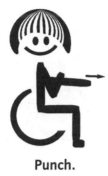

Punch.

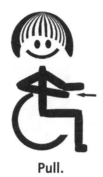

Pull.

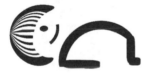

Swing.

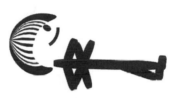

Hug.

Bend.

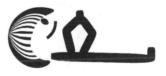

Push.

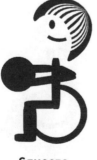

Squeeze.

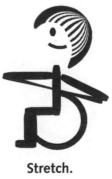

Stretch.

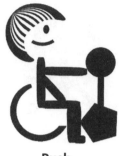

Push.

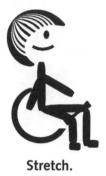

Stretch.

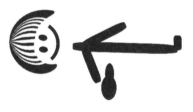

Squeeze.

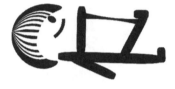

Stretch.

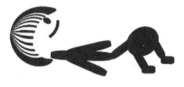

Push.

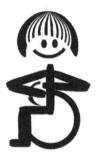

Roll.

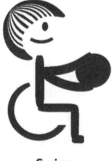

Swing.

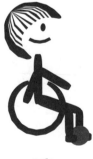

Lift.

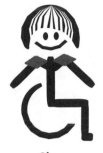

Shrug.

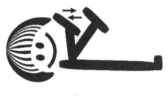

Squeeze.

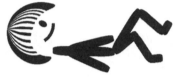

Stamp.

Clap.

PARTNER BODY ACTIONS

Dodge.

Clap.

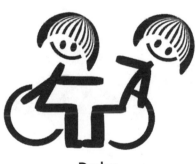

Push.

Lift.

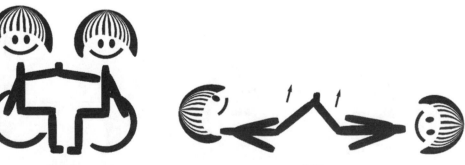

Bend.

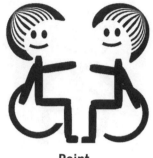

Point.

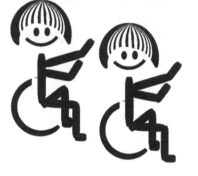

Climb.

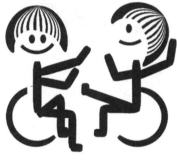

Dance.

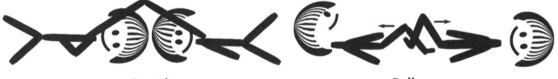

Stretch.

Pull.

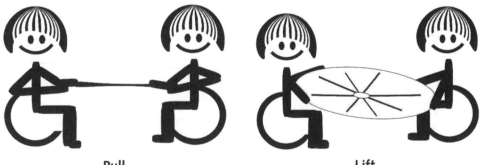

Pull.

Lift.

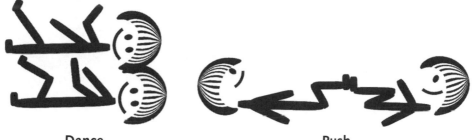

Dance.

Push.

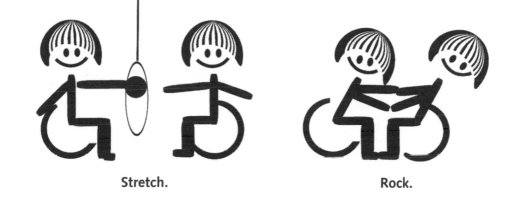

Stretch.

Rock.

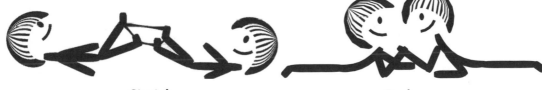

Stretch.

Push.

2

DROP

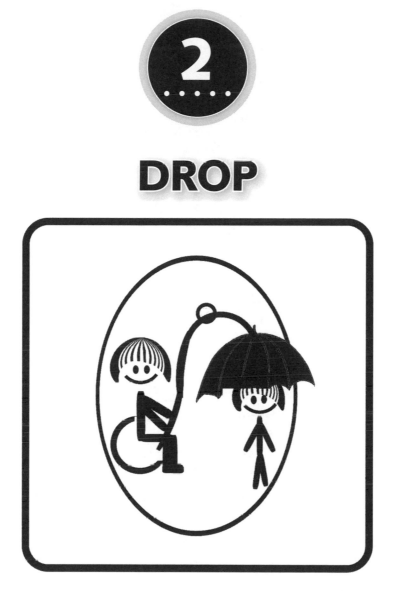

One day I tied several small parachutes to ropes and hung them from the ceiling. Participants had a chance to hold the ropes and then let the parachutes drop. The group sang "Drop Goes the Weasel" as they paraded around the room, passing under the parachutes. Each time the group sang "drop," the parachutes came down, covering the players. They loved it. I loved that William, who had shown no connection to or interest in any activities, actually came into the room the next day, looked for the parachutes, and then went to stand under one . . . waiting . . . with a big smile!

A drop involves releasing an object that is being held stationary by, or on, one or more body parts. Application of force is not necessary. A very simple way to drop an object is to balance it on a body part and then move the part until the object falls off.

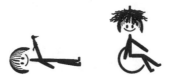

Another way to drop an object is to place it in the hand or fingers and work to release it.

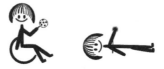

A drop can also be done by wedging a soft ball or other object between two body parts and releasing it.

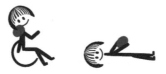

Use balls that are easy to grasp when teaching drop. These can include sponge balls, yarn balls, squishy balls, semi-inflated balls, or foam balls.

Any object can be used for dropping activities. Place a puppet or pom-pom loosely on a hand so that it is almost falling off. Ask the participant to move his hand until it falls off. That's dropping! Items can be dropped from almost any body part. As an attention getter, drop an object that makes noise.

To hang a ball for any activity, place it in a mesh bag (even the kind oranges and onions come in) and suspend it, using string or rope, from anything available. Use chinning bars, basketball hoops, soccer nets, or the ceiling. It works best to have a way to adjust the height of the suspended object so each person can be accommodated.

If you hang balls from the ceiling, use sturdy eye screws. If the ceiling is suspended, use plant hooks (available in the plant section of most stores). The plant hooks clip to the grids between the ceiling tiles.

INDIVIDUAL DROP

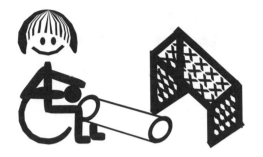

Into the tube.

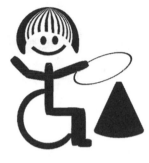

Over the cone.

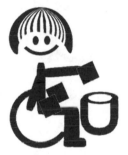

Beanbag in the bucket.

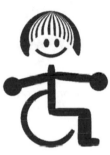

Two at a time.

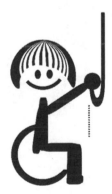

Lift and drop.

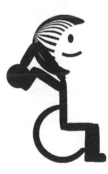

Back drop.

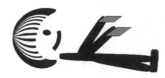

Drop two at a time.

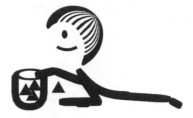

Shape lift and drop.

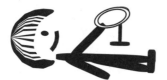

Ring drop or toss.

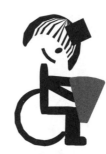

Off the head and into the cone.

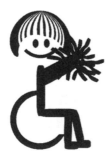

Pom-pom lap drop.

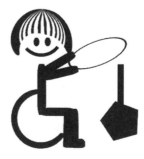

Over the tee.

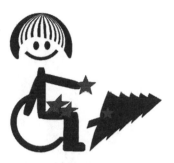

Decorate the tree.

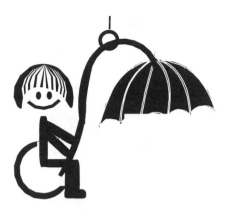

Parachute-on-a-rope drop.

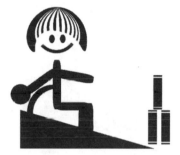

Drop on the wedge.

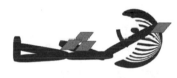

Over-the-head drop.

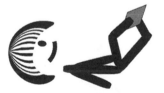

Foot drop.

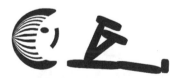

Noisy rhythm sticks.

PARTNER DROP

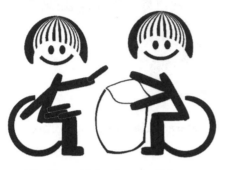

Rhythm sticks in a ball bag.

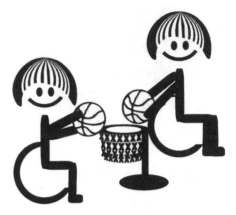

Basketball drop.

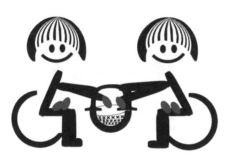

Plastic eggs in a basket.

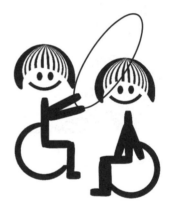

Human hoop drop.

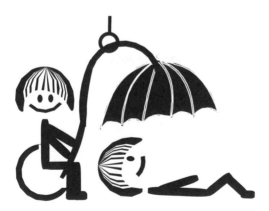

Parachute-on-a-rope drop
on a friend.

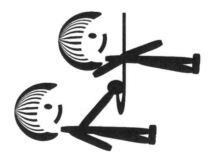

Alternating lift and drop.

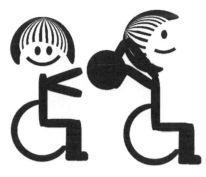

Duo back drop.

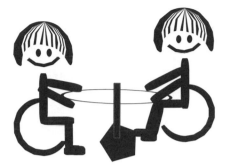

Cooperative hoop drop.

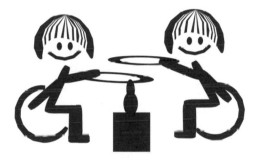

Who goes first?

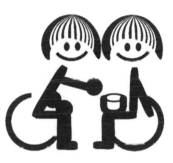

A drop in the bucket.

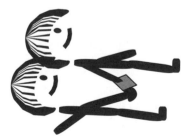

Partner palm drop.

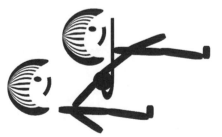

Cooperative lift and drop.

3

PUSH

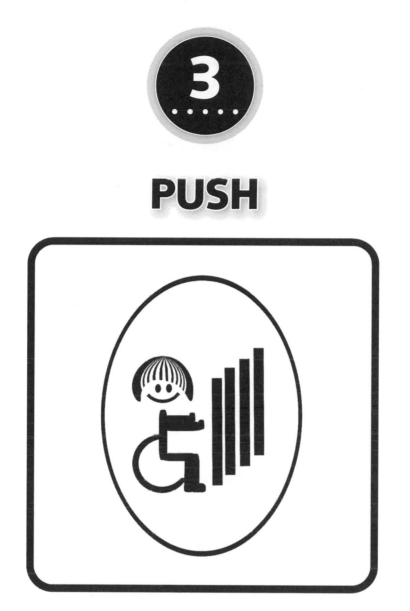

One day I asked Mary to push a folded mat that was standing on end. This mat was lined up with several other mats, all placed on end close to one another. Her soft push brought the first mat into the second, the second into the third . . . and so on! Soon the entire class couldn't wait for a turn to push.

A push involves applying force to move an object away from a person. A push can be as simple as an arm movement in the appropriate direction, even if the object does not move.

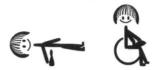

A push can be a sideways sweep, a small forward movement, or even light contact with an object.

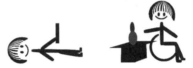

Any body part can be used for a push.

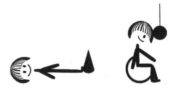

Any application of force, no matter how small, can be considered a push.

To be motivating, an activity must be fun and grab the attention of the participant. Objects that make noise, that return to the player, that fall down, that will move easily, that can be stacked—these can all be motivating.

A push is the start of a throw, and in some cases will be the only way a participant can get an object moving. If a participant's grasp is weak or nonexistent, a push *is* a throw.

Modify games such as Ping-Pong or air hockey for using a push and a larger, lighter object, such as a balloon. Make a game table by placing an open mat on a stack of mats or on the arms of strategically placed wheelchairs. Both options allow participants to be closer to the game. If the table is too long for playing lengthwise, play widthwise.

INDIVIDUAL PUSH

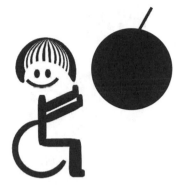

Swinging ball.

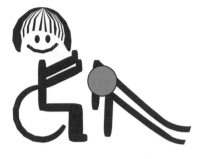

Down the ramp.

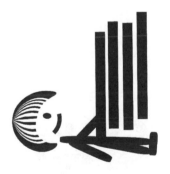

Shuffleboard push.

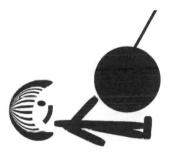

Swinging ball.

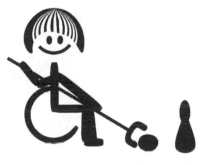

Domino mats.

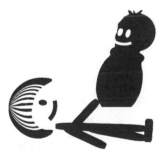

Bop bag push.

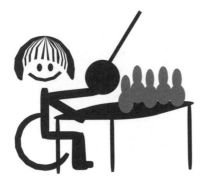

Skittle bowling.

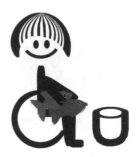

Fish in a bucket.

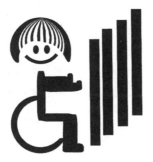

The domino effect.

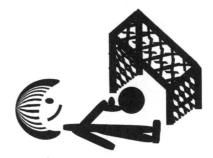

Air hockey ball push to the net.

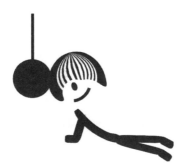

On-the-belly head push.

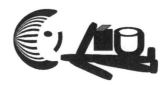

Off the box and into the bucket.

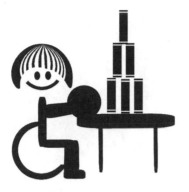

Table push.

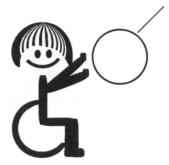

Hoop push.

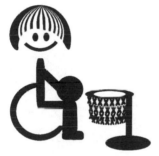

Lap push into the basket.

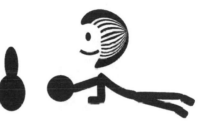

A ball at a pin.

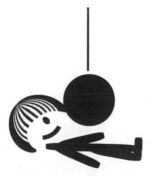

Heading the ball.

Push belly out on inhale.

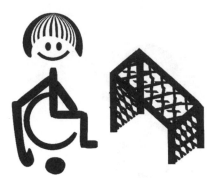

Hockey push.

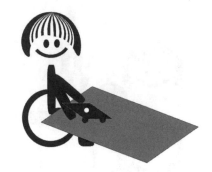

Scooter down the mat.

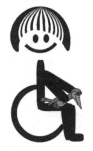

Puppet off the lap.

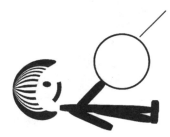

Hoop push.

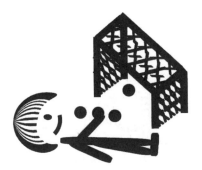

How many? net push.

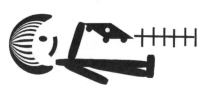

Scooter push for distance.

PARTNER PUSH

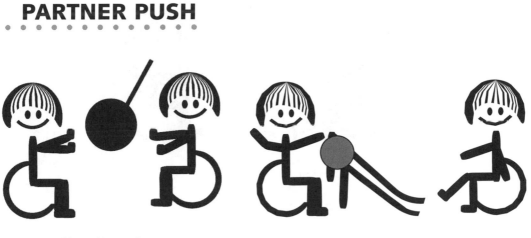

Keep it moving.

Push and trap.

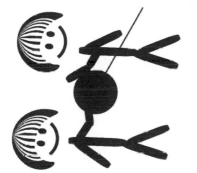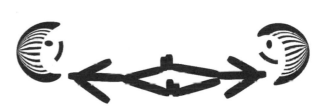

Partner push.

Foot push.

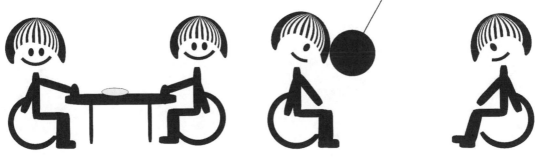

Air hockey.

Head to head.

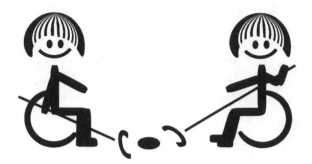

Shuffleboard push.

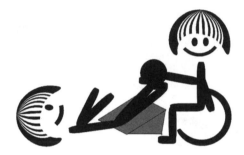

Push-down-the-legs catch.

4

TOSS

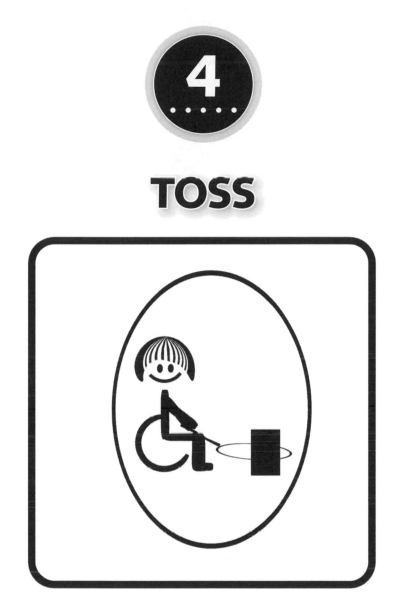

As part of our County Fair unit, we played a game called Lasso Challenge. The game called for a hula hoop to be tied to a rope and tossed over a cardboard box. Jeremy not only roped the box, but he then proceeded to pull it across the floor to his chair. His grin told us all how pleased he was.

A toss involves finding a way to gently project an object into space. In its simplest form, a toss can be balancing an object on the hand or arm and moving it into the air with minimal application of force.

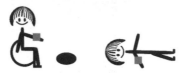

A toss can also be a simple motion, such as a fling, that moves an object from the hand or arm into the air.

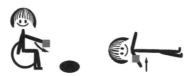

A toss is simply a gentle throw. Why differentiate? A toss requires less force than a throw. In throwing, an increase in speed and force is encouraged. In a toss, a gentler motion is called for. It is another way to teach the movement components of force and speed. As in throwing, it matters little if the toss is underhand, overhand, or sidearm.

In teaching the toss, tie a rope or string to objects to be tossed or thrown to make retrieval easy.

In both teaching and practice activities, emphasize a slow, smooth movement. The variations of movement in each person may be small. After initial trials, encourage a slower and softer movement to project the object. Use verbal cues such as "slow" or "easy."

Mix the activities of toss with those of throw by placing targets or other activity components closer for toss and higher or at a greater distance for throw. Use verbal cues to help participants distinguish the difference in the movements.

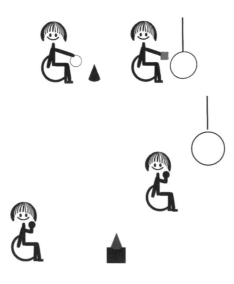

INDIVIDUAL TOSS

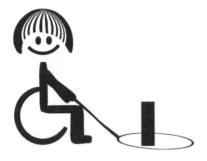

Hoop-on-a-string lasso toss.

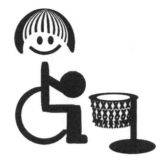

Basketball toss.

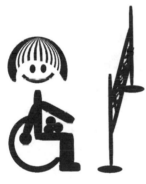

Over-the-net toss.

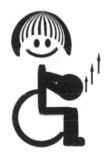

Higher and higher.

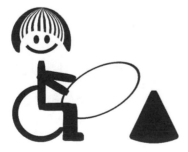

Hoop toss.

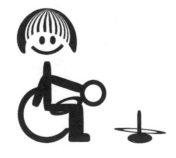

Ring toss.

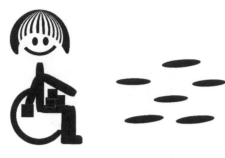

Beanbags on the circles.

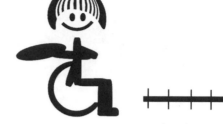

Flying disc toss for distance.

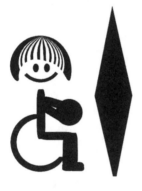

Wall toss and catch.

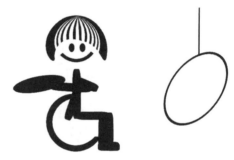

Flying disc toss.

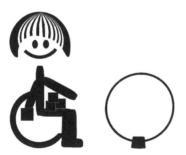

Beanbag toss.

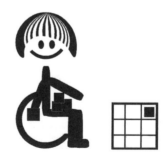

Tic-tac-toe toss.

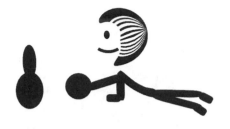

Ball-at-a-pin toss.

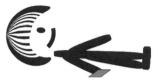

Over-the-belly toss.

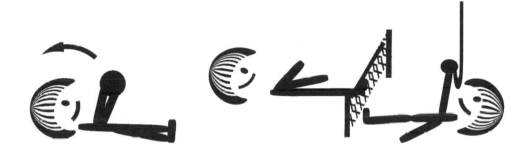

Two-hands-over-the-head toss.   **Over-the-net-on-a-string toss.**

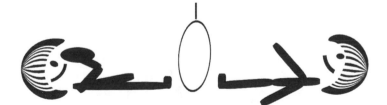

Football-through-the-hoop toss.

PARTNER TOSS

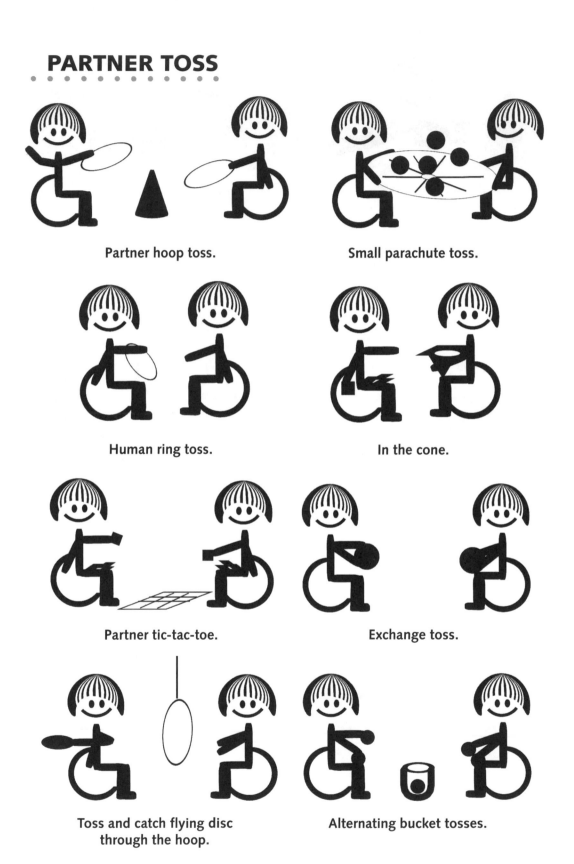

Partner hoop toss.

Small parachute toss.

Human ring toss.

In the cone.

Partner tic-tac-toe.

Exchange toss.

Toss and catch flying disc
through the hoop.

Alternating bucket tosses.

5

THROW

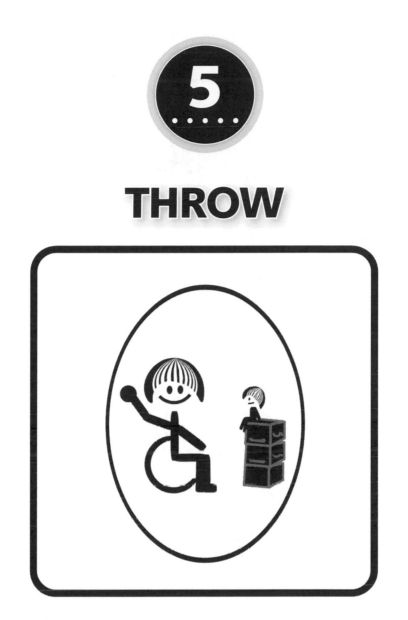

Emmy never did anything independently and never seemed to smile. I placed a small doll on top of a stack of cardboard building blocks and threw a ball at the blocks. The blocks tumbled down, and so did the doll. Emmy started to laugh and promptly picked up a ball, indicating she would like to try. She threw over and over, laughing every time the doll fell to the floor.

A throw involves finding a way to project an object into space using one or both arms. In its simplest form, a throw is applying force to nudge or push an object into space.

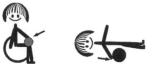

A throw can be a simple application of force when releasing or moving an object.

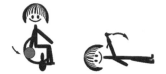

Throwing requires some experimentation to see what works best for each person. Participants can throw overhand, underhand, or sideways, using one hand or two. Try them all; it makes no difference. A push may be a throw for some participants. When grip strength is weak or nonexistent, try the following:

1. Use a soft ball (such as a Nerf ball) and place it in or on the participant's hand. Ask the player to fling or shake the ball loose. Place the ball so it can be easily moved, putting just enough of the ball into the hand to keep it in place.

2. Use a Wiffle ball and place a finger a short way into one of the holes. Shake it off.

3. Place a ball or other object between two hands, arms, or wrists. Ask the participant to find a way to release it.

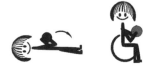

Provide step-by-step verbal directions and initial hand-over-hand assistance with each spoken direction. Gradually reduce the physical assistance and keep the verbal cues consistent. Use simple cues such as "Up, throw," or "Lift, throw."

After a participant's basic method of throwing is established, the skill can progress by increasing the speed or force of its execution. Use verbal cues such as "Throw faster" or "Throw harder."

Place targets close to the participant, especially at first. Select targets that invite participation; try items that are colorful, noisy, huge, or silly. Ask players to try to hit *you* with the ball. Fall on the floor when they do!

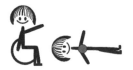

Post a picture of a favorite staff member or a famous person as a target. Hang pictures of lions and go big-game hunting. Be creative!

INDIVIDUAL THROW

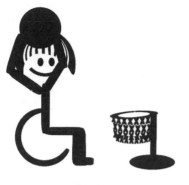

Over the head.

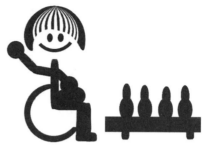

Overhand.

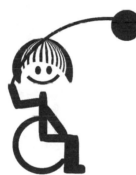

Overhand on a string.

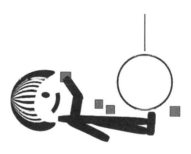

Through the hoop.

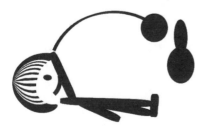

Ball on a string.

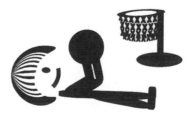

Two points!

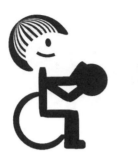

At the wall.

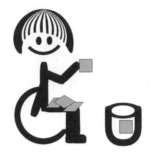

In the bucket.

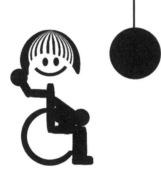

At the hanging ball.

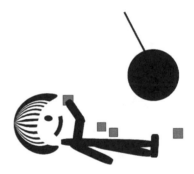

At the swinging ball.

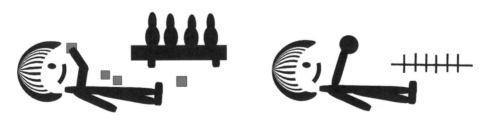

Pick 'em off.

Throw for distance.

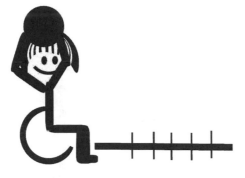

Throw for distance.

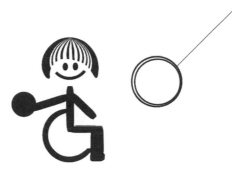

Through the swinging hoop.

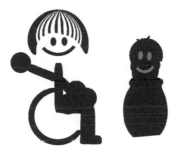

At a bop bag.

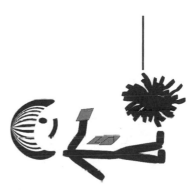

Hanging pom-pom.

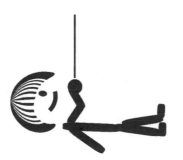

Ball on a string.

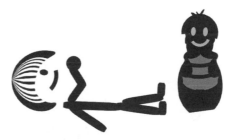

Velcro vest on a bop bag.

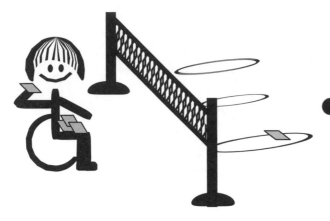

Over the net into the hoops.

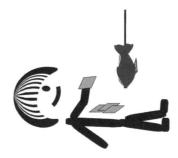

Knock the ball off the tee.

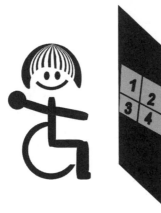

Velcro target.

Beanbags at a fish.

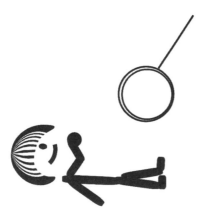

Through a swinging hoop.

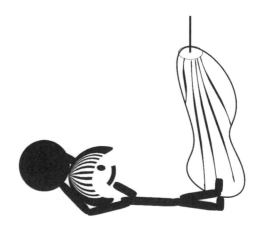

At a hanging parachute.

PARTNER THROW

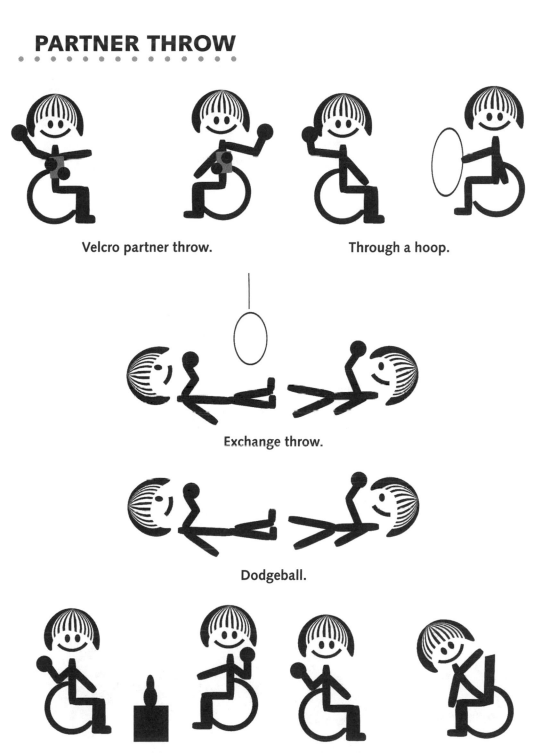

Velcro partner throw.

Through a hoop.

Exchange throw.

Dodgeball.

One . . . two . . . three . . . GO!

Throw and dodge.

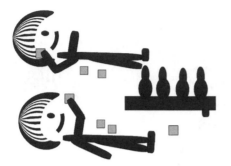

Partner pin throw.

Block the throw.

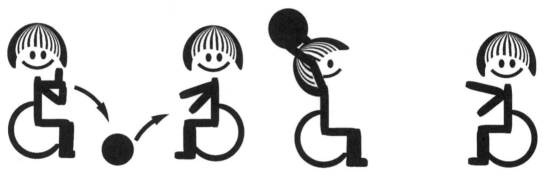

Bounce pass.

Over-the-head pass.

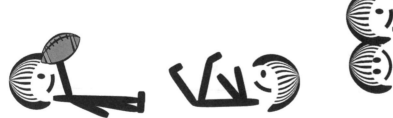

Through-the-legs pass.

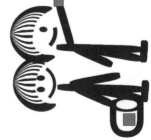

Over a friend into the bucket.

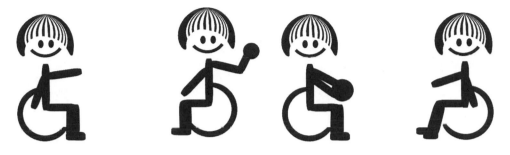

One-hand throw and catch.   Throw and kick.

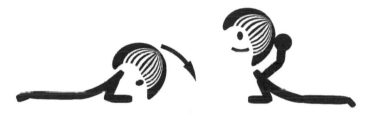

Throw and duck.

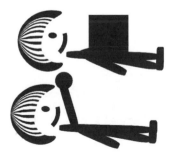

Knock the box off.

6

KICK

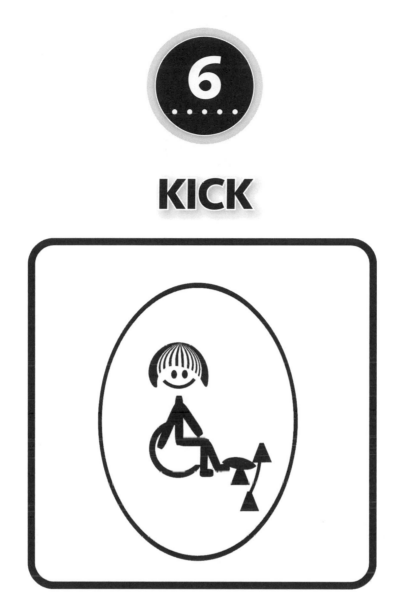

I design football games so that staff can provide help in most of the game play. Participants have two actions to do independently. The first is to hike the ball to start play. The second is to score the extra point or field goal. The goalposts are two cones connected by a rope. Moving the cones nearer to or farther from each other allows you to adjust the height of the "crossbar" to meet individual needs. The distance to the cones is also adjusted for each player. During one game, Ronnie was to kick the extra point. Excitement was high since the extra point would win the game. He normally kicked by moving his legs enough to allow a ball placed on his feet to fall away. This time the wheelchair footplates were removed, and the ball was placed on a cone very near his feet. Ronnie managed to move his legs enough to make contact with the football, which then dropped over the rope and scored the winning point.

A kick involves applying force to move an object using one or both feet. In its simplest form, a kick can involve moving one or both feet enough to shake off or dislodge an object that has been placed on or between the feet.

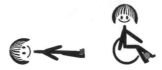

A kick can also start with light contact or a soft push with one or both feet.

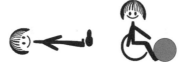

A kick can also begin by placing an object on the wheelchair footplates and having the participant move it with the feet. To tip the scales in the player's favor, use on object that can be placed so it is partially hanging off the footplates.

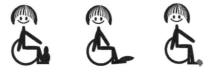

As with other skills, after the foot has made initial contact with the object, encourage the participant to apply more force or speed. Use a verbal cue such as "Kick *harder*" or "Kick *faster.*"

Always tip the scales in favor of the participant:

1. Use an object that can be moved easily, such as a punchball or a balloon.

2. Use an object such as a puppet, beanbag, or pom-pom that can be placed so it is practically falling of the feet before any movement has been made.

3. Place the object against the feet so any movement will make the object move.

Find a way for each participant to be successful. Provide initial assistance when needed. For instance, you might say, "I am going to help you move your foot. See how that feels? Now you try it." Several repetitions may be needed for the player to find the muscles involved in the action. Allow plenty of time for the participant; do not be in a rush.

What if a participant cannot move his legs at all? Place an object in front of the wheelchair and let the participant (or a helper) wheel the chair into the object and move it. That, too, is a kick.

The greatest gift you can give a participant is time to figure out what to do and how to do it.

INDIVIDUAL KICK

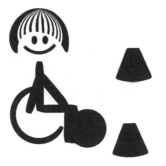

Through the cones.

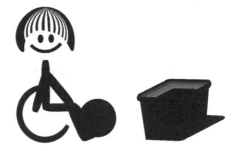

Into the box.

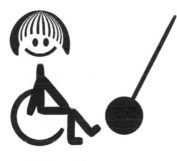

Kick on the move.

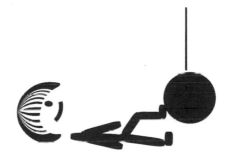

Progressive kicks (one kick, then two kicks, then three kicks . . .).

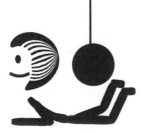

Belly kicks.

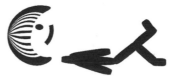

Alternating kicks (right, then left, then right . . .).

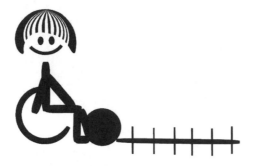

Kick for distance.

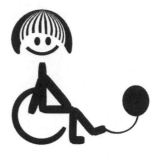

Punchball kicks.

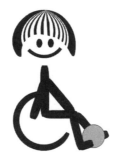

Let go!

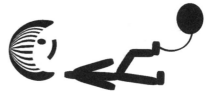

Punchball kicks.

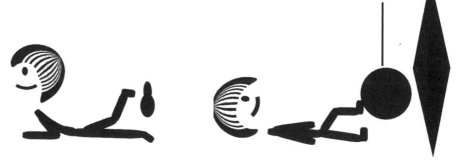

Pin kick.

To the wall.

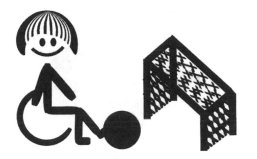

Into the net.

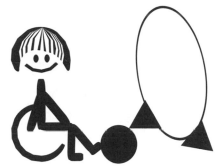

Through the hoop.

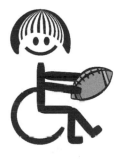

Drop kick.

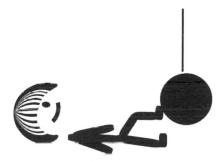

A hanging ball.

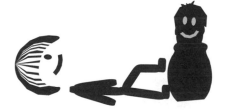

Back atcha.

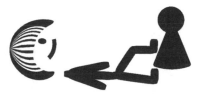

A ball off a cone.

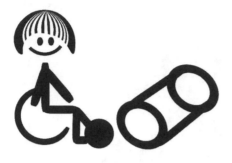

Through the tunnel.

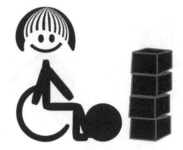

Knock 'em down.

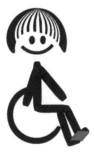

Beanbag off the foot.

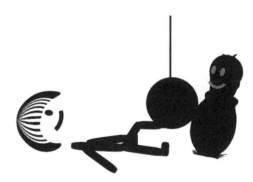

A ball and a bop bag.

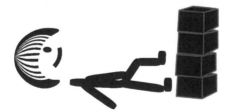

Knock 'em down.

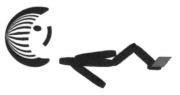

Beanbag off the foot.

PARTNER KICK

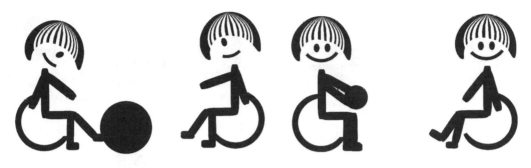

Partner kicks. Toss and kick.

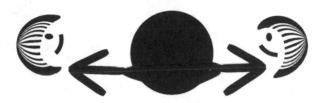

The great kickoff.

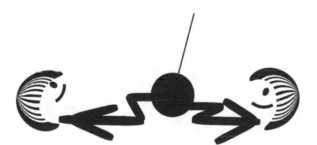

Ball kick.

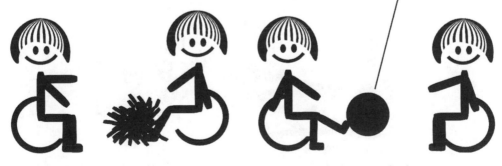

Pom-pom kick and catch. Alternating kicks.

Strike or spare?

Toss and kick.

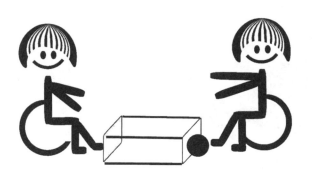

Through the box.

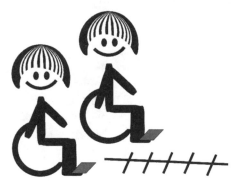

Beanbag-off-the-foot kick
for distance.

Partner beanbag kick and catch.

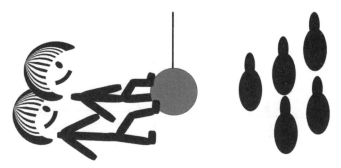

Partner kick bowling.

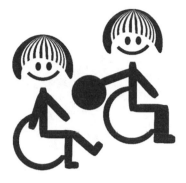

Drop and kick.

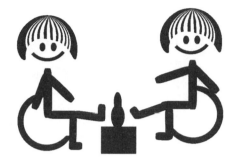

Kick contest.

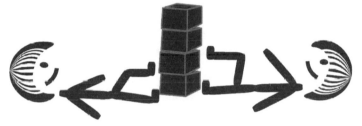

Take turns.

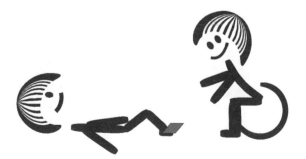

Kick up and catch.

7

CATCH

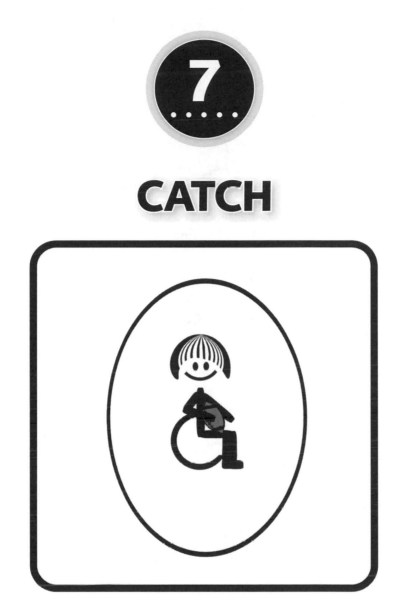

In one slightly chaotic football game, Annie was to catch a pass. She was prompted to raise her arms and then bring them down when the ball hit her lap. Unfortunately, the ball hit her lap and began to bounce off. No one knows just how she did it, but Annie managed to scoop the ball with one arm onto her other arm and keep it there, scoring the winning touchdown! Sometimes, the excitement of play can lead to the unexpected.

A catch involves finding a way to stop an object as it moves through space and maintain control of it. A catch can involve using one or both arms to capture an object that has been gently tossed onto the lap.

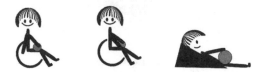

A catch can also be a hugging action, clasping a ball or other object to the chest as it approaches. Toss softly at the chest in the beginning.

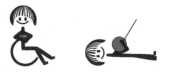

You can help a player catch an object by using Velcro paddles, mitts, or vests. In the beginning, toss the ball directly to the Velcro prop.

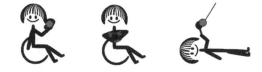

A participant can use a foot or both feet to catch (trap) the object.

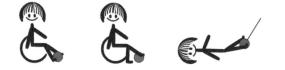

Practice with a stationary ball at first. Place it on a lap or hang it from a string and work on capturing the ball with the arms or hands.

Any object can be used to teach catch. Think in terms of items that will stay put, such as a puppet or a pom-pom, and that allow the participant time to move arms or hands into position. A semi-inflated ball, or one that can be compressed a bit, will be easier to catch than fully inflated or bouncy ones. Very light balls such as punchballs or balloons are harder to catch. Use an object or ball that will easily stay in place.

A hanging ball or other object will allow the addition of a slow swinging motion. Adjust the height of the hanging ball to accommodate the participant's range of motion. Remind participants to keep their eyes on the ball. Use a verbal cue such as "Arms ready . . . catch."

INDIVIDUAL CATCH

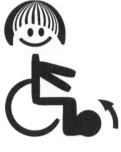

Lift and catch.

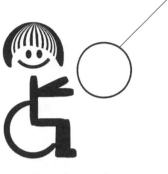

A swinging hoop.

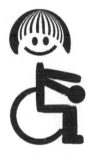

Hand to hand.

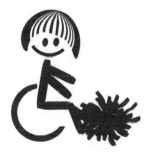

Pom-pom catch.

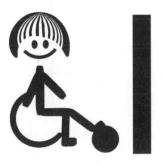

Wall rebound trap.

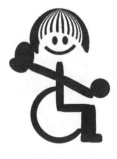

Velcro mitt.

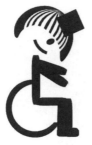

Beanbag-off-the-head catch.

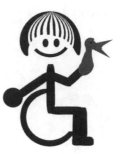

Puppet catch.

Bounce catch.

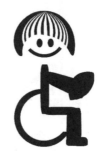

Football toss and catch.

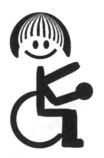

One-hand catch.

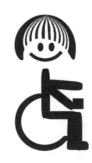

Beanbag toss and catch.

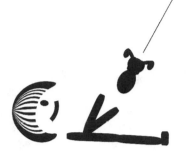

Puppet on a string.

Pool noodle on a string.

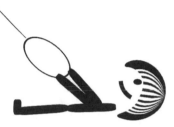

Hoop on a string.

PARTNER CATCH

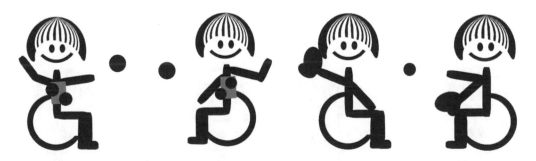

Velcro vest catch.

Velcro mitt doubles.

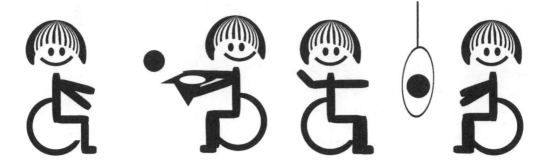

Cone catch.

Through-the-hoop catch.
(Try adding Velcro mitts!)

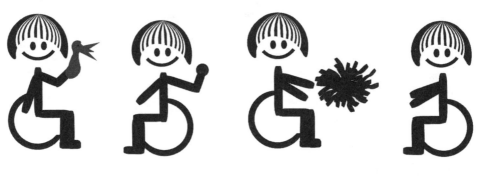

Puppet partners.

Pom-pom partners.

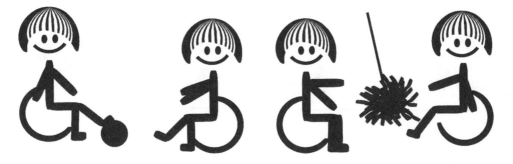

Kick and trap.

Pom-pom kick up and catch.

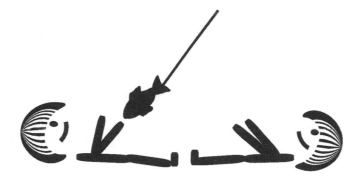

Catching fish.

Two-arm catch on a wedge.

8

STRIKE

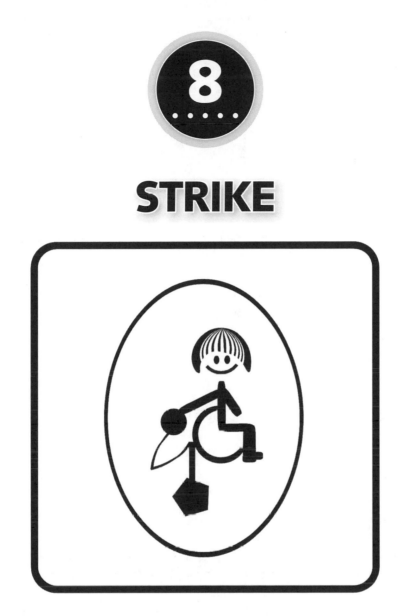

Jimmy, who has multiple disabilities and very limited movement, managed to move his arm repeatedly to strike a punchball. He was in his wheelchair, facing, and quite close to, a wall. The punchball was tied to a batting tee by a string. He repeatedly moved his arm enough to contact the punchball as it came back from the wall. It was hard to tell who was more excited that day: he or I!

A strike involves contact between two objects with some degree of force. A strike can begin as a simple contact between a body part and an object and progress to a push with the selected body part.

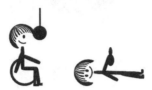

A strike can also involve one object making contact with another and then progressing to deliberately using one object to push another.

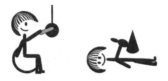

Start by using objects that can be easily moved. A punchball balanced on your hand near the participant's hand or arm is a good way to start. A punchball is light enough to move with very little force applied.

Use objects that are easily moved. If necessary, allow the object to touch the body part being used for the striking action. Raise or lower hanging objects to meet the participant's range of motion.

After initial trials, encourage the player to apply more force or speed to the action. Use verbal cues such as "Strike *harder*," or "Strike *faster*."

Start striking activities by using the body parts that have the most ability to move. Add equipment after the striking action has been practiced. Many objects can be a bat: a dowel rod, a rhythm stick, a paper towel tube. The bat can be light, fat, thin, short, or long. Choose equipment combinations that make for success.

INDIVIDUAL STRIKE

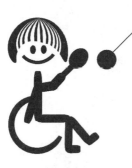

Paddle strike.

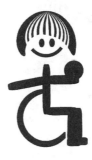

Sidearm strike.

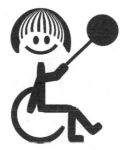

Punchball strike.

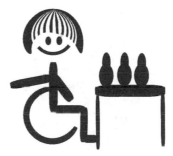

Sidearm pin strike.

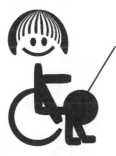

Low strike.

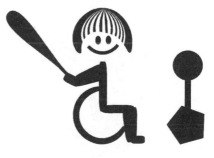

Baseball strike.

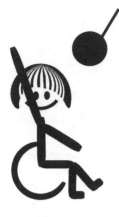

High strike.

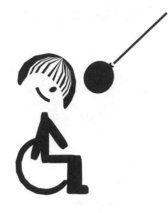

Head strike.

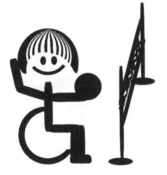

Serve.

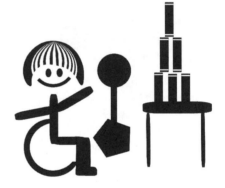

Knock 'em down.

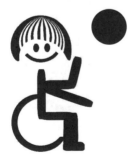

Toss and strike.

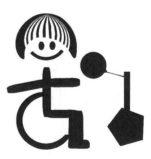

Repeated strikes.

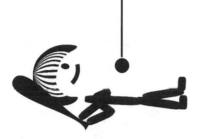

Bat and ball.

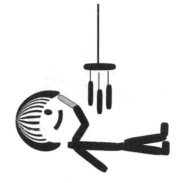

Rhythm stick and wind chimes.

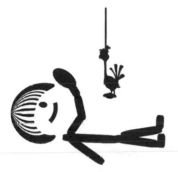

A paddle and a chicken.

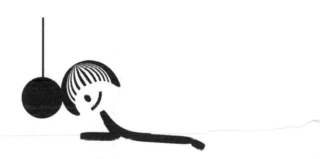

Head strike.

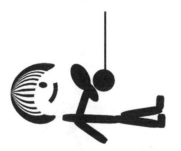

Plastic bowling pin and a ball.

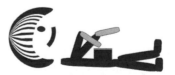

Belly drumming.

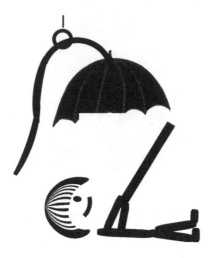

A noodle and a 'chute.

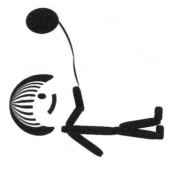

Punchball strike.

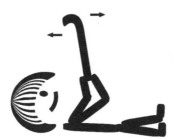

Air hockey.

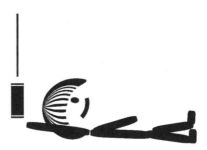

Stretch 'n' strike.

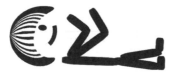

Karate strikes in the air.

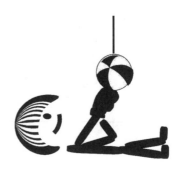

Beachball punch.

PARTNER STRIKE

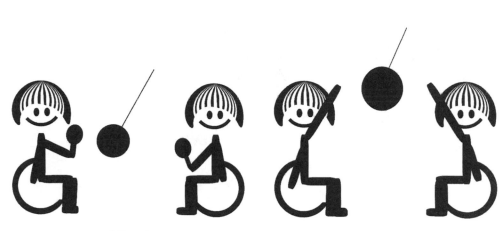

Paddle play.

Stretch 'n' strike.

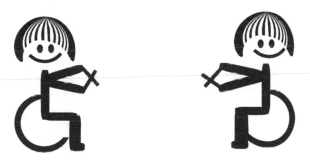

Rhythm stick copycat.

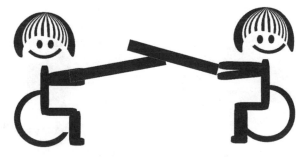

Noodle fencing.

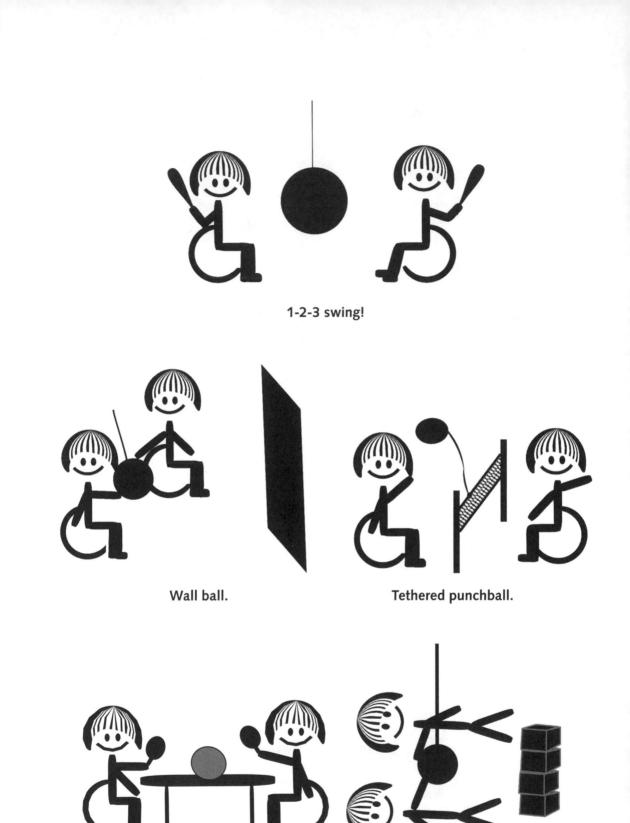

1-2-3 swing!

Wall ball.

Tethered punchball.

Tabletop balloon ball.

Ready, set, go!

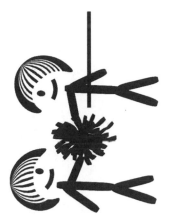

Alternating pom-pom strikes.

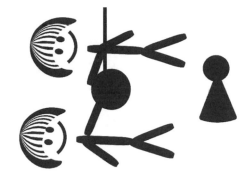

Ready, set, go!

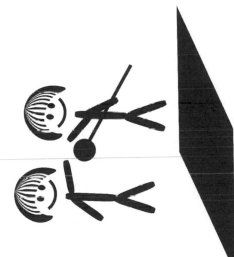

Supine handball.

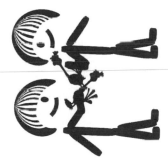

Rubber chicken fight.

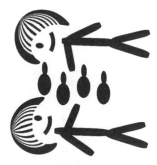

Knock 'em down.

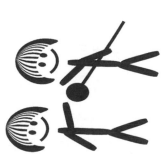

Wall baseball.

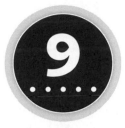

ODDS AND ENDS

One summer I decided to introduce some offbeat ideas with my students. Jousting quickly became a favorite: Players held pool noodles (or noodles were attached to their wheelchairs), and recordable devices (such as a "big mac") were also attached in a prominent place. On "GO!" participants moved across the room, each trying to use the noodle to touch the recordable device, which was programmed to say "Ouch, ouch, ouch" when hit.

Sometimes an idea for an activity sparks another activity idea. Sometimes activities help develop less obvious skills or competencies. Sometimes activities are just for fun. This chapter includes all those types—activities that were afterthoughts, activities that didn't fit elsewhere. Activities should be fun, stimulate the desire to participate, and bring a greater personal awareness to the individual. Whether that awareness concerns the body, the breath, or the mind is immaterial. It is wonderful to realize you can enjoy physical activity when you have limited physical capabilities, to meet challenges you never thought you could. Even if you will never run a 50-yard dash, throw a ball across the room, or kick a field goal in a competition, there is a lot you *can* do.

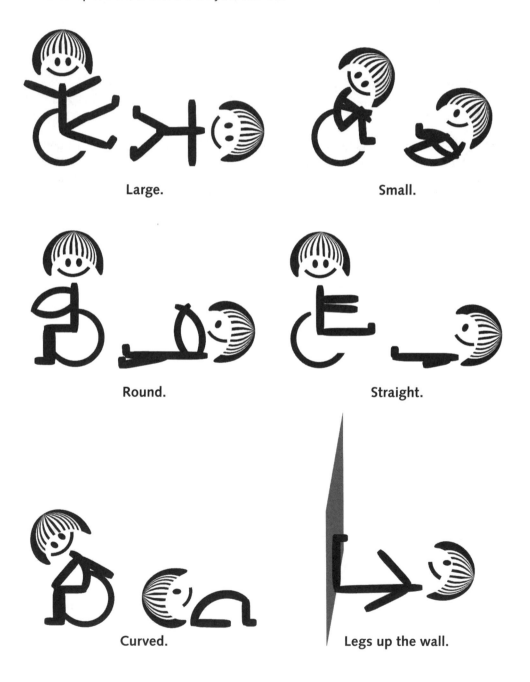

Large.   **Small.**

Round.   **Straight.**

Curved.   **Legs up the wall.**

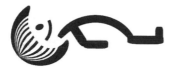

Chest lift.

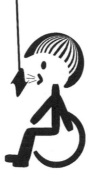

Tissue blowing.

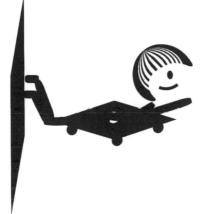

Scooter push off the wall.

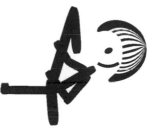

Low bar pull-up.

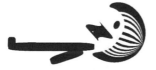

Tissue blow off the face.

Chicken toss and catch.

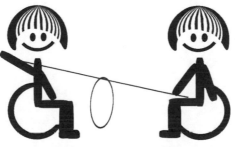

Ring-on-a-string exchange.

10

GAMES

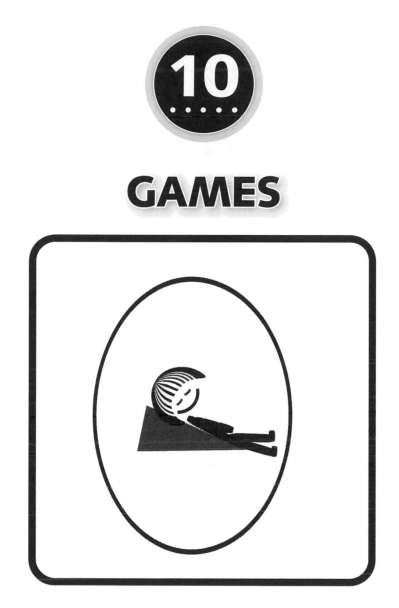

One way to play Red Light, Green Light is for all participants to be on the floor. At the words "green light," everyone except for the player designated as *It* moves in place in whatever way is possible. With eyes closed, *It* (or someone else) counts to 10. At 10, *It* calls, "Red light," opens his eyes, and tries to catch anyone who is still moving. One day, Hank, a new class member, was chosen to be *It*. At that time I had little idea of Hank's cognitive abilities, but I knew that his physical abilities were quite limited. I explained open eyes and closed eyes by covering Hank's eyes with my hand and then taking it away. Once I knew he understood, we started the game. As soon as I said, "Green light. Close your eyes," Hank did so and kept them closed until I said, "Red light. Open your eyes." The game was repeated several times with Hank opening and closing his eyes at the appropriate time. I believe Hank was as happy as I was with his ability to participate on his own in some way. Teach your players what they should do and then give them the opportunity to try it.

A game is a multiplayer activity that has a goal, a method of play, and an outcome. At its simplest, it's an activity in which several players follow the same overall guidelines to reach an objective.

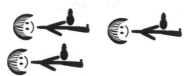

Be the first to knock over your pin.

Games and their objectives should be simple, and the rules should be kept to a minimum.

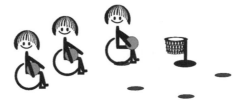

Be the first to make a basket from each of the spots on the floor. Once you make a shot, move to the next spot. If you miss, the next player takes his turn.

Vary the skill used in the game in ways that best allow each person to meet the objective. Hints and ideas for personalizing participation are found in the Options section of each game description.

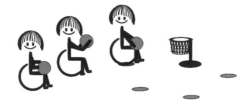

Push, throw, or toss.

Select appropriate props (such as a lighter ball, an extended handle, an oversized target, and so on) for each individual in order to facilitate participation.

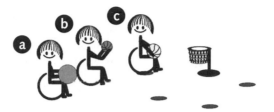

(a) Larger, softer ball; *(b)* lighter, smaller ball; *(c)* regular-size and -weight ball.

Adjust space requirements to meet each person's capabilities. Move game items closer, higher, or lower. Decrease or increase the distance to be traveled.

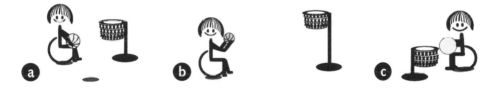

(a) Regular setup. *(b)* Higher, greater distance. *(c)* Lower and closer.

In all games there should be at least one part that expects, and works toward, independent participation. Look at games to determine where a player could most easily perform independently. The action should be modified to meet the individual's capabilities.

Push a ball to another player, or a helper, to hike.

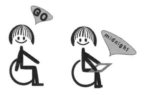

Incorporate players' verbal skills when possible; program a communication device that players can use if they are nonverbal.

Hold a ball close to, in the lap of, or touching a player to put or keep it in play.

Push or drop a ball out of the lap and on to the base to make an out.

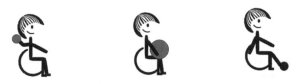

In chase games, if mobility is limited, use a ball to tag players. Toss, throw, push, or kick the ball to tag another player. Contact with the wheelchair also counts as a tag. Use a *soft* ball.

An activity needs to be repeated several times to work out the glitches for each person. Never judge the success or failure of an activity after just one, two, or even three tries.

BEANBAG RACE: CHAIR VERSION

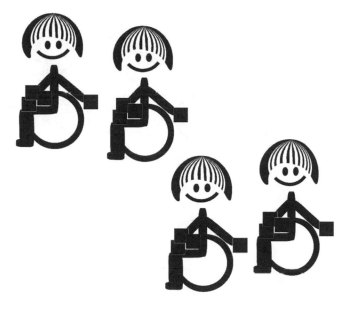

Objective

Be the first person to drop all your beanbags on the floor.

Play

Provide the players with beanbags, the same number for each player. On your signal, all players drop their beanbags, one at a time, to the floor. The player who finishes first is the winner of each round.

Options

- If the group is large, arrange for a word or signal to announce when a player has finished.

- For those with limited grasping ability or minimal arm movement, a helper can place the beanbag on the player's arm. The player then shakes or moves her arm until the beanbag falls off.

- If a participant is unable to grasp, she could also push the beanbags from her lap one at a time.

BEANBAG RACE: FLOOR VERSION

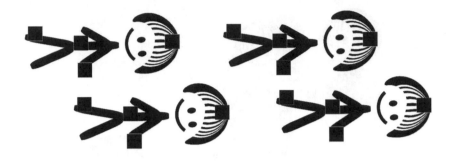

Objective

Be the first person to get all your beanbags on the floor.

Play

Place beanbags on various body parts. Each player should have the same number of beanbags in approximately the same places. On your signal, players work to get all their beanbags onto the floor. The player who finishes first wins each round.

Options

- Arrange a signal or sound to indicate being finished if the group is large.
- Place the beanbags in such a way that they can be shaken or wiggled off the body parts.
- In cases of very limited mobility, the beanbags may need to be placed so they are already partially off the body when play begins.
- This game can also be played with participants lying on their bellies.

PINBALL

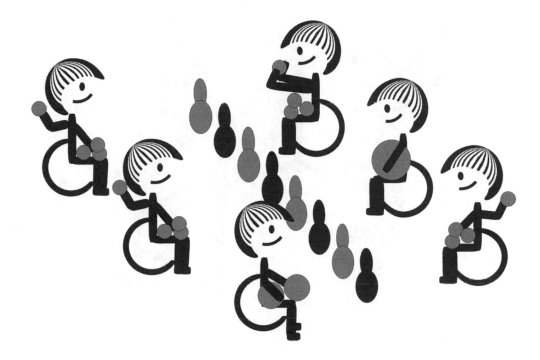

Objective

Be the first team to knock down all your team's pins or to have the most pins down when all the balls have been used.

Play

Set plastic bowling pins in two colors, or with identifying marks, in a line on the floor. Alternate colors or marks. Choose two teams and assign each team pins of one color or mark. Give each team an equal number of balls. On your signal, all the players throw, toss, or push their balls at the pins, trying to knock down those of their own team. If a player knocks down a pin from the other team, it stays down. The first team to knock down all their pins is the winner. If all the balls have been played and there are still pins standing, the team with the most pins down wins.

Options

- Place wheelchairs closer to the pins if necessary. All wheelchairs do not have to be the same distance from the pins. Distances should be modified to meet the abilities of each player.
- Balls can be pushed off the lap or a wheelchair tray and rolled to the pins.
- Use balls of differing sizes and weights to afford each player the best degree of independent play.
- If enough help is available, the game can be played until all the pins are down. Helpers retrieve the balls that have been used and return them to a player, keeping the action going until all the pins of one team are down. Assign the same number of helpers to each team.

PUNCHBALL VOLLEYBALL

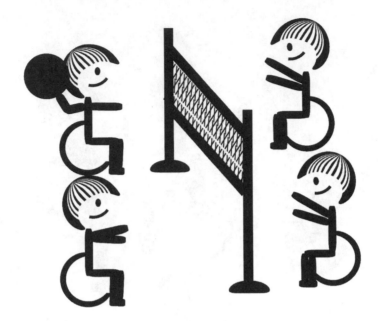

Objective

Score more points than the other team in a limited time.

Play

This game is played like regular volleyball. The serving team retains the serve and scores a point each time the ball hits the floor on the other side of the net. When the ball hits the floor on the serving side of the net, the serve moves to the other team. A team scores points only when serving. The serve can be from anywhere on the court. Rotating players after a serve is optional. The serve can be given to any player no matter where he is on the court.

Options

- If the ball is not in a player's reach when it comes over the net, or after contact by a team member has been made, staff can assist by bringing it to the closest player.

- Provide hand-over-hand assistance only when needed. Most players, including those with extremely limited mobility, can make a punchball or balloon move.

- If the ball is not hit hard enough to clear the net, other players or staff can give an assist. Determine ahead of time how many assists are allowed before turning the ball over to the other team. Three is the standard number.

- Add excitement by having staff be a part of the action. Require them to keep the ball in motion using small taps as they bring it to a player. If they drop it, it's side out!

A DIFFERENT CHARLIE OVER THE WATER

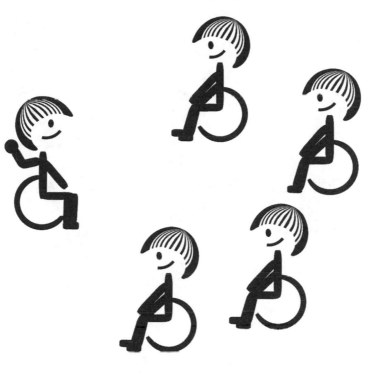

Objective

Tag a player before she can place her hands on her knees or perform another action. (In chase and tag games, throw a soft ball to tag the players.)

Play

One person is chosen to be Charlie and given a soft ball. Other participants are placed in a semicircle around Charlie. Everyone who can speak, including staff, chants, "Charlie over the water, Charlie over the sea. Charlie caught a blackbird, but he can't catch me!" When the chant is ended, all players perform the chosen game action, for instance, placing their hands on their knees. Meanwhile, Charlie tries to tag players before they can complete the action. Charlie tags a person by hitting her or his chair with a *soft* ball. If Charlie is successful, the tagged player chooses a new player to be Charlie. If Charlie does not tag a player, he gets two more turns to try. After three tries, he chooses another player to take his place.

Options

- Use a ball that is appropriate to each person who takes a turn as Charlie.
- The ball can be thrown or pushed. It can be rolled to hit a chair.
- Place participants within a reasonable distance of each player who takes a turn as Charlie.
- Choose body parts or actions that can be done by players but present a small challenge.
- If necessary, staff can help players throw the ball or perform the action.

As in all assisted activities, constant communication is a must between participant and staff. Time must be allowed for the individual participant to attempt the activity.

HOW MANY BEFORE: CHAIR VERSION

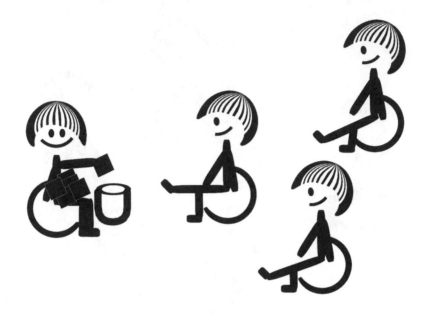

Objective

Drop as many beanbags (or other objects) into the bucket as you can before the other participants complete the designated activity.

Play

Provide one player with a supply of beanbags and a bucket. Choose an action the group must complete. On your signal, each member of the group begins to perform the designated activity. At the same time, the player with the beanbags begins to drop them into a bucket. When all participants have completed the activity, action stops, and the beanbags in the bucket are counted. Keeping score is optional. A new beanbagger is then chosen, and play is repeated with another activity. Participants can take turns choosing the movement or exercise to be done.

Options

- Beanbags can be pushed, dropped, thrown, or moved in whatever way possible to get them toward the bucket.
- The bucket should be placed to accommodate the ability of the beanbagger.
- The beanbags can also be dropped on the floor as an alternative to using a bucket.
- Allow performance of the action to be adjusted according to individual abilities. In the previous example, a leg lift could be anything from just moving the foot or leg to a full leg lift. Always modify the performance to meet the capabilities of the individual, even in group activities.

HOW MANY BEFORE: FLOOR VERSION

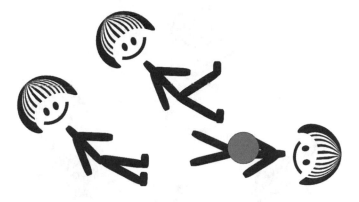

Objective

Move a ball or other object from the belly as many times as possible while the rest of the group completes the designated activity.

Play

Place a ball or other object on the belly of a designated player. Choose an action that the group must perform. On your signal, each member of the group begins to do the chosen activity. At the same time, the designated player begins to wiggle or move in any way possible in an attempt to move the ball from his belly. When the ball or other object falls to the floor, the player, or a helper, picks it up and replaces it on the belly and again tries to dislodge it. When everyone has completed the activity, action stops, and the number of times the ball has been moved off the belly is announced. Keeping score is optional. Repeat the game with a new player to move the ball, or other object, from his belly.

Options

- Use a ball appropriate to the individual: smaller, larger, softer, and so on.
- Choose activities that are doable for everyone. Participants can take turns choosing the activity.
- Substitute other actions for moving the ball from the belly. For example, a player could count how many times he could tap a hanging ball or kick it with his feet.

> *Be creative; it's more fun!*

HIT AND RUN

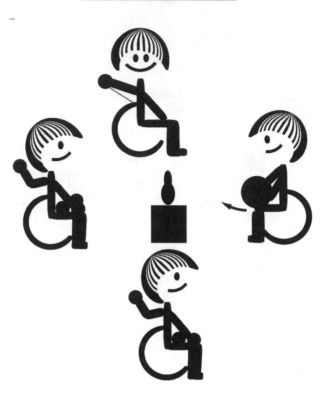

Objective

Be the first to knock down the bowling pin.

Play

Place a bowling pin on a table or other flat surface. Each player has several balls or beanbags. On your signal, everyone tries to hit the bowling pin and knock it down. The first player to knock over the pin takes one lap around the circle of players, scoring one run. Play is repeated. If the pin is still standing after all the balls or beanbags are thrown, the pin scores a run. Retrieve the balls and beanbags and play another round. After several rounds, announce who won the game: The players or the bowling pin.

Options

- Use just one ball per player and attach it to the wheelchair with string so the player can retrieve the ball independently. If you are using this option, play can continue until the pin is down, and players can score runs personally rather than as a group.
- When necessary, provide assistance in throwing or in taking the lap around the circle. Remember to communicate with the player and leave plenty of time for the player to perform as independently as possible.
- Space chairs for success; some may need to be closer to the pin than others.
- The pin can also be placed on the floor, allowing some players to push a ball from their laps instead of throwing it.

KICK BOWLING

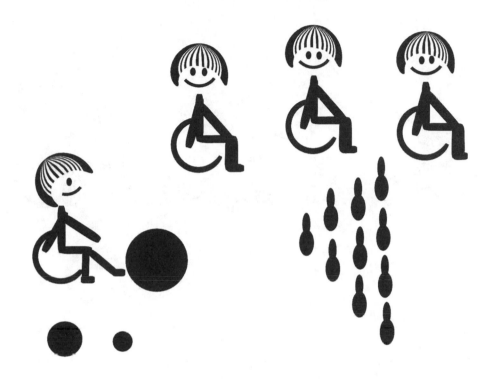

Objective

Kick the ball and knock down as many pins as possible in two tries.

Play

Set up pins in a standard bowling pin formation. Players have two tries to kick the ball and knock over as many pins as possible. Play and score as in regular bowling. Use two teams, or play as one group and keep individual scores.

Options

- Make the size of the ball appropriate to the individual's ability to kick.
- Modify the distance to the pins to allow for a successful turn, even if it means placing the chair right in front of the first pin.
- When mobility is very limited, the ball can be placed on the player's feet and moved off in any way possible.
- This is a good inclusion game. For those with normal kicking ability, use a small ball or increase the distance to the pins. For those with limited abilities, use a very large ball or shorten the distance to the pins.

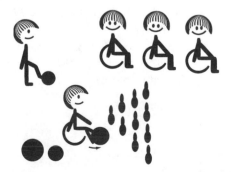

GONE FISHING

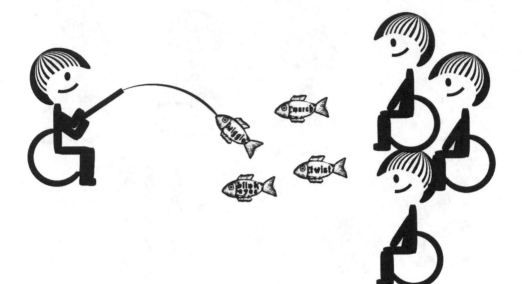

Objective

Catch a fish and lead the group in the activity printed on the fish.

Play

Create a fishing rod by attaching a length of string with a magnet on one end to a dowel. Cut fish from card stock and add a steel paperclip to each one. Write a different activity on each fish. Each participant takes a turn catching a fish and then leading the group in the indicated activity for a designated amount of time. Give enough time for the group to actually do the activity to the best of their ability. Have a "catch and release" policy.

Options

- Use several fishing poles and see who can catch a fish first.
- As an alternative, make many fish and play for a period of time to see who can catch the most fish.
- An alternative method of play is to drop or toss beanbags onto fish.
- A player can also push a ball from his lap and let it roll to, or over, a fish as an alternative way of catching the fish.

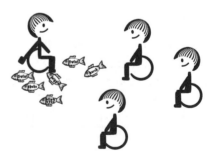

IN GOOD TIME

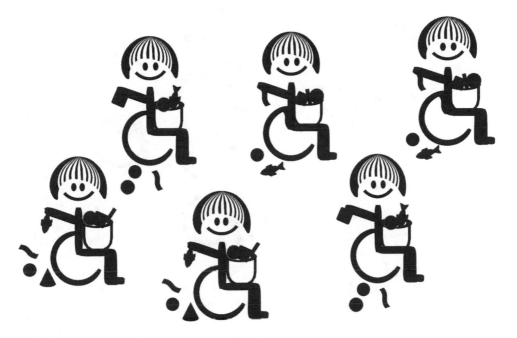

Objective

Drop items from the bucket onto the floor in a fixed time.

Play

Fill buckets with beanbags, small balls, small stuffed animals, rhythm sticks, and more! On your signal, all participants try to drop as many objects on the floor as possible in the time allowed. At the end of the time period, the player with the most objects on the floor is the winner.

Options

- Use objects suitable to the grasping skills of the participant.
- For easier grasping, use squishy or soft balls, or even a sponge. Sponges make great items to use in activities. Trace figures (such as animals, letters, or numbers) on them and cut them out. This allows you to tailor the items to the skills of the player. Leave a long narrow part to grasp, or put a hole in the center. Any shape and embellishment that will provide help when grasping can be used.
- A participant can touch an item if grasping is difficult, and a helper can then put it on the floor.
- A shoebox, plastic bin, or any container with easy access can be used in place of a bucket.

> You can change the rules! Anything that works and is safe is acceptable. Find activities and ways to participate that are within the capabilities of the players. These can be different for each one. It doesn't matter. What matters is that everyone is able to participate as independently as possible.

WHAT'S THE NUMBER? CHAIR VERSION

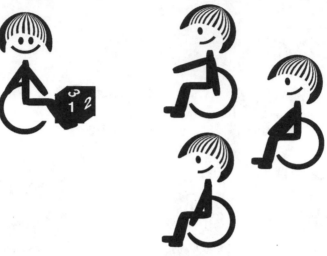

Objective

Kick the box and, using the number key, perform the indicated activity.

Play

Any square box can be used for this game. Put a number on each of the six sides. Make a chart that shows what activity matches each number on the box.

1 = Wiggle for 10 seconds.

2 = Rock side to side 5 times.

3 = Nod your head 3 times.

4 = Clap your hands and make a noise.

5 = Stretch your arms wide and hold them there for 3 seconds.

6 = Stamp your feet 10 times.

One player kicks the box, and then all players participate in performing the activity indicated by the number shown. Choose a new kicker after each activity.

Options

- Use the large, soft dice often sold in auto stores and seen hanging on rearview mirrors.
- If a player cannot kick independently, place the box on her feet. She then moves her feet or legs until the box falls to the floor.
- The box can be placed on a cone or other object to bring it to a level that allows a player to kick more easily.
- Participants who can kick easily should have the box placed relative to their range of motion when kicking.
- A skill besides kicking can be used to move the box. Use push, drop, toss, or any other movement that you would like to develop.
- A different approach can be to have players balance the box on a body part and try to hold it steady for several seconds before letting it fall to the floor. Try putting it on the head, knee, shoulder, back of the hand, and so forth.

WHAT'S THE NUMBER? FLOOR VERSION

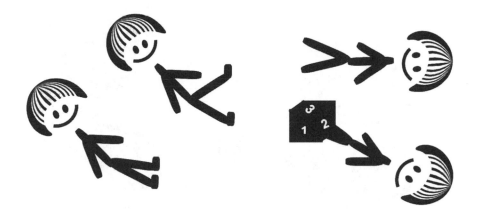

Objective

Move the box off of a body part and, using the number key, perform the indicated activity.

Play

Make a box and a chart as in the preceding version of the game. Place the box on a player's body part, such as an arm, leg, torso, or knee. The player then moves the part of the body the box is on until the box falls to the floor. All participants then perform the activity corresponding to the number displayed. At the end of the activity, choose a new player to be It. Allow plenty of time for participants to do the indicated activity.

Options

- Place the box on weaker areas of the body to motivate movement. Make it a challenge—one that's not too hard but not too easy!
- Choose some activities, such as rolling over, pushing backward, or lifting the head and shoulders, that are unique to the floor.
- Have players try the game (or any other floor versions of games) while lying on their bellies or sides.
- As in the chair version, an alternative way to play is to place the box on a body part and have the player try to balance it there for several seconds before letting it fall to the floor.

COOPERATIVE BALL PUSH: CHAIR VERSION

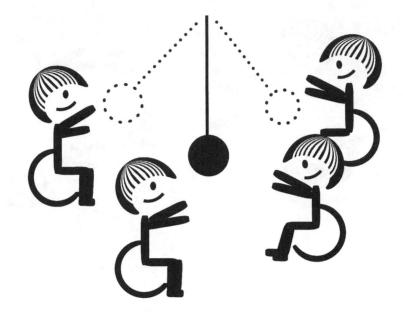

Objective

Keep the ball moving for as long as possible.

Play

Attach a ball on a string to something stationary overhead. Circle the players around the ball and start the ball swinging. Players push the ball as it swings near them. Count the number of successful pushes before no one can reach the ball. Announce the number of pushes and begin another round, trying to beat the previous count. Any contact with the ball is a push.

Options

- Set a number of pushes that the group will try to reach. If the group reaches that number, they win; if not, the ball wins. Keep score!
- Use old-fashioned jump rope chants, counting the number of pushes instead of jumps. Or make up your own chant: "Wiggle and giggle, sit up tall. How many times can you hit the ball? One, two, three, four . . ."
- Use a very large ball and a small circle to increase the chance of success.

COOPERATIVE BALL PUSH: FLOOR VERSION

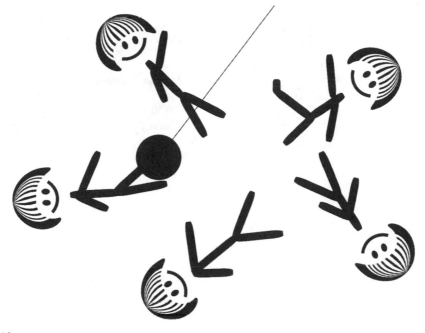

Objective

Keep the ball moving for as long as possible or to reach a designated number of pushes without a miss.

Play

Suspend the ball overhead from a stationary object. Players lie on the floor with the ball within reach. Players push the ball as it moves toward them. Count the number of successful pushes. In the next round, have players try to beat the number. You can also give players a specified number of pushes to make. If the group makes the goal, they win. If not, the ball wins. Keep score!

Options

- Any contact with the ball can be considered a push.
- Allow any body part to contact the ball: foot, arm, head, hand, and so on.
- The ball should be suspended at a level that accommodates the player with the smallest range of motion.
- Use a ball that is large enough to reach and move easily. A large beach ball in a net bag or tied to a string works well. Beach balls come in sizes up to 36 inches (90 cm) and sometimes more.
- Substitute other objects for the ball, such as a ball bag filled with newspaper, or a bird puppet (players must keep the bird flying). Use objects that are safe for the participants.
- Add a paddle or short bat for each player to use to keep the ball moving by striking it rather than pushing.
- Equipment must accommodate the needs of the players. Equipment is a tool, a means to an end. Use whatever works!

KNOCK IT DOWN RELAY: CHAIR VERSION

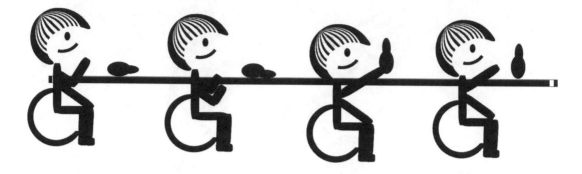

Objective

Be the first team to knock down your pins.

Play

This game is run like a regular relay race, with one team member completing his turn before the next can go. However, in this case the players remain stationary. Choose two teams. Position each team near a counter, table, or stack of mats. Place one plastic bowling pin on the table or counter next to each player. On your signal, each player in turn knocks down his pin. The first team to complete the action wins the race.

Options

- Pins can be placed on top of a cone or box next to each player.
- Pins can also be placed on the arm of a wheelchair. If they tend to fall off, place them on a soft beanbag for support, or use a bit of adhesive putty or masking tape to help anchor them lightly.
- Place the pins on the player's dominant side. Or, if using the counter or table, place the wheelchair so the player can access his dominant side.
- Pins should be placed to accommodate each individual's range of motion.

KNOCK IT DOWN RELAY: FLOOR VERSION

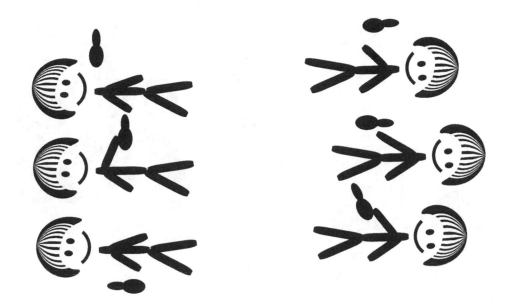

Objective

Be the first team to knock down your pins.

Play

Choose teams and have them lie on the floor in two lines. Place a pin within reach of each player. Play as a regular relay race; each team member must knock down her pin before the next player can start.

Options

- Place pins on the player's dominant side and close enough to accommodate her range of motion.
- Use pins that are light enough to be easily moved.

HOOP PASS RELAY

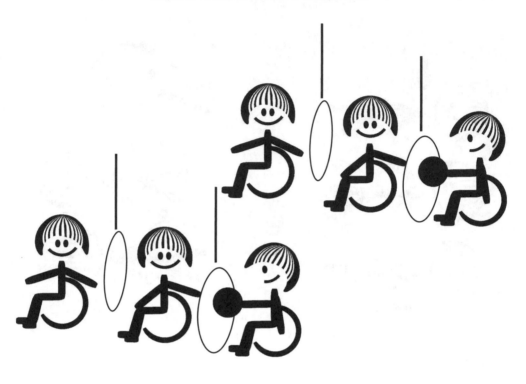

Objective

Be the first team to complete passing an object through a hoop from one player to the next.

Play

Hang two sets of hoops from the ceiling by string or rope. If hanging them is not possible, use hoop stands. Place the hoops at heights appropriate for the players. Choose two teams. On your signal, the first player on each team passes the object through the hoop to the second player, who in turn passes it to the next player until it reaches the end. The team which finishes first is the winner.

Options

- Use an object that is easily handled.
- Place chairs close enough to the hoops that players do not have to overstretch.
- Make arrangements for retrieving the object in case it falls to the floor.
- If the ability to grasp is an issue, play as a simple tagging game. Participants must reach through the hoop and tag the next player. This option also works well when range of motion is limited.
- This race can be done without any hoops. Players simply pass an object down the line.
- Instead of using hoops, connect a rope or string to cones. Players pass the object under the string.

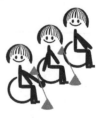

LAP RELAY

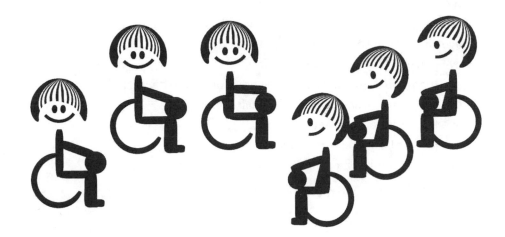

Objective

Be the first team to move a ball from the lap of each player.

Play

Choose two teams. On your signal, each player takes a turn moving the ball, in whatever way possible, from his lap. When the last player has moved the ball from his lap, the race is over, and the team that finished first is the winner of the race.

Options

- If players have severe limitations, the ball can be placed under the hand or arm. The arm or hand should then be moved in whatever way is possible to release the ball.

- If a player has difficulty reaching his lap with his hands, place the ball in his lap and allow any movement to be used that will make the ball drop.

- The ball, held in place by the player's arm or hand, can also be placed on the arm of a wheelchair instead of the lap.

- Use other objects in place of a ball. Use items that a person can move easily.

Need more ideas for relay races? Most of these will work in the chair or on the floor.

- Have players use their feet to knock pins down.
- Lay a pin on the player's belly or lap. Wiggle it off.
- Place a pin on the nondominant side of a player and have her reach across the body to knock it down.
- Have each team member pass a pin to the next player. The last player has to set it on the floor and knock it over.

(continued)

LAP RELAY *(continued)*

- Place a pin near a player's head and she can use a head motion to tip it over.
- Use a different object in the race. Substitute a pom-pom on the player's belly, lap, or head.
- Have the player pick up and set down a ball using the feet.
- Have each player shake a beanbag off a body part.
- Have players blow a tissue off their faces.
- Have them tap a rhythm stick on the floor, or on the counter, three times.
- Ask them to roll over or twist in the chair a few times.
- Have them stamp their feet five times.
- Have players blink their eyes three times.
- Have them push balls to knock over, or hit, a target.

Determine what actions and movements are possible and go from there.

BALL DANCING

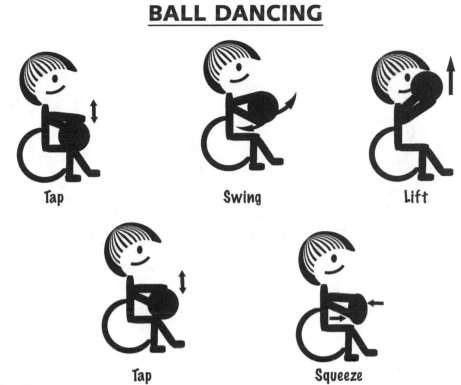

Tap   Swing   Lift

Tap   Squeeze

Objective

Move the ball to the music in a variety of ways.

Play

Play music with a clear beat or sing a familiar song using your own words. Have the players move a ball in different ways in time with the music. Use some, or all, of the pictured movements, depending on the music. Add more movements, or more repetitions of simple movements, as needed. The song "Alley Cat" works well, as do the suggestions in the options section of this activity.

Options

- Use a ball sized for the individual. In addition to a regular ball, you can use a pom-pom, a squishy ball, a partially inflated ball, or any object that can be easily moved.
- Players who cannot grasp an object can perform the motions without a ball, using their hands or arms.
- Try this activity with the song "If You're Happy and You Know It." Substitute your own words (such as "If you're happy and you know it, tap the ball"). Another classic song that works well is "Here We Go Round the Mulberry Bush." Use actions that suit the activity instead of the song's original lyrics.
- Allow individual actions to be as independent as possible, even if they have to be changed or modified.
- Create actions that can be done by those participating.

Ensure that participants can perform activities to the best of their abilities.
The idea is to get all players participating in some way on their own!

DROP THE FLAG

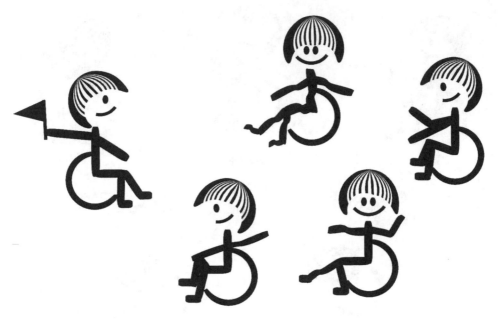

Objective

Keep moving until the flag hits the floor. When the flag hits the floor, all movement stops.

Play

One player holds the flag. On your signal, all the other participants begin to move in any way possible. When the person with the flag drops it, everyone must stop moving by the time the flag lands on the floor. Identify those who stopped moving in time and then choose a new flag holder.

Options

- When the ability to grasp is an issue, place the flag on a body part and the player shakes or wiggles until the flag falls to the floor.
- Instead of having players move until the flag hits the floor, try giggling. Everyone must stop giggling when the flag lands (this is *hard*!).
- Another option is to choose a specific nonlocomotor movement for participants to perform until the flag lands on the floor.
- For a greater challenge, add a period of time after the flag hits the floor during which players must hold still or keep from giggling. A few seconds or a count to five is usually sufficient.

TEAM EXCHANGE

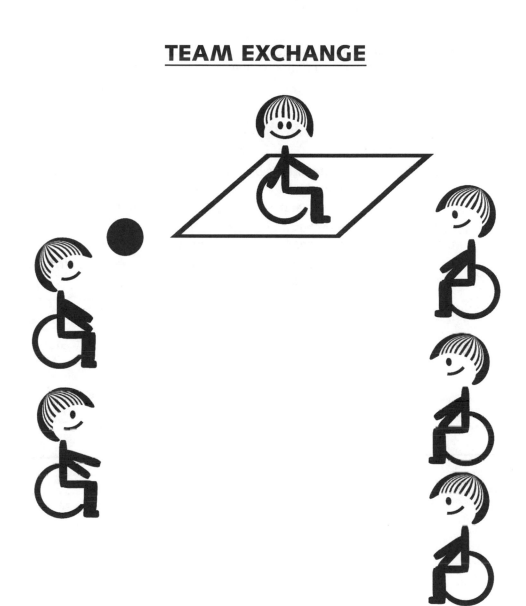

Objective

Have the most players on your team at the end of the play period.

Play

Choose two teams. Place chairs next to each other in a line, one team facing the other. Team A has three tries to use a ball to tag a player, or the player's chair, on the opposite team. If team A is successful, the tagged player moves to a designated area. If not, the ball goes to the other team and play begins again. When a player is tagged, his team has a chance to get him back by performing a task, chosen by the opposite team, within a certain time limit. If successful, the player is returned to his team. If not, the player must join the opposite team and play continues, with team

(continued)

TEAM EXCHANGE *(continued)*

B trying to tag a player on the opposite team. Play continues by alternating teams. At the end of the play period, count the number of players on each team. The team with the most players wins.

Options

- To tag another player, the ball can be thrown, pushed, kicked, rolled, or pushed from a wheelchair tray.
- Tasks should be appropriate to the abilities of the players. Modify the performance required for each team member.
- You can write tasks on paper, and a team member can choose one.
- To add another element to the game, place papers with tasks written on them on the floor and let a team member toss a beanbag to choose one.
- Vary the size of the ball used to meet the capabilities of the players. Use anything from a tennis ball to a *huge* ball.

REACH FOR HEIGHT

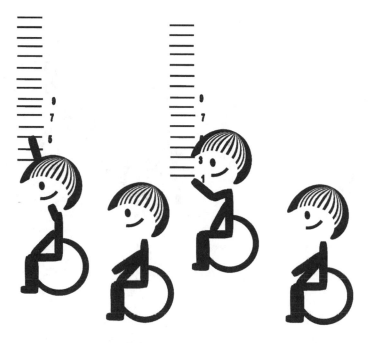

Objective

Increase the distance each player can stretch.

Play

Create a measuring chart with equidistant lines and post it on a wall. Each player reaches as high on the chart as possible, and the distance reached is recorded. Each player then reaches again, trying to increase her distance. Repeat three times and take the best distance. The player who improves her stretch the most (calculated by subtracting the smallest stretch from the greatest) is the winner of each round. Repeat using the opposite arm.

Options

- Make the lowest line on the chart low enough on the wall so every player can reach.
- Mark distances in small increments.
- Position wheelchairs to facilitate the reach of each player.
- Use this activity as one event in a series of activities or as a stand-alone activity.

Remember, it's about the experience, not the competition!

WHAT'D I SEE

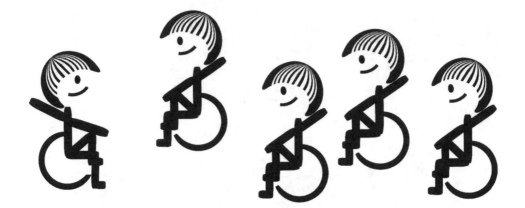

Objective

Identify which movements to copy and which to ignore.

Play

This activity is played like the traditional Simon Says game, but with different words spoken in a rap music rhythm. The player who is the rapper makes various movements, each preceded by saying, "What'd I see? You doing like me?" The other participants copy the movement. When the rapper says, "Do like me," instead of "What'd I see? You doing like me?" participants hold the previous movement rather than copy the new one. Those who do the new movement are identified, and a new rapper is chosen from those who did not change. Allow every player to have a turn as rapper.

Options

- Pair nonverbal participants with another player or staff member to work as a team.
- Program communication devices to speak for the participant.
- Try this game on the floor! Remember that games on the floor can be played on the belly or the back.

> In games that use spoken words, staff can speak for nonverbal participants. As always, staff should maintain a meaningful connection to the participants they are helping. Communication devices can also be programmed or game overlays made so the individuals can be verbal.

A NEW HAPPY AND YOU KNOW IT:
<u>CHAIR VERSION</u>

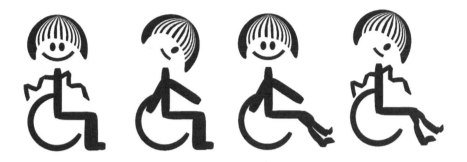

Objective

Create new and different actions to a familiar tune.

Play

Play an instrumental version of the song "If You're Happy and You Know It," or sing without music. Each participant takes turns making up a movement for one of the verses in the song. Everyone does the movement at the appropriate point in the song.

Options

- Use movements easily manageable for the group.
- If a participant cannot think of a movement, note whatever he is doing (such as smiling, shaking his head, making a face) and quickly say the words to fit that action. Let everyone copy the participant's action.

Note: In musical activities such as this, the repetition of each verse allows extra time for a player to do the action. For example, in the traditional version, all would clap their hands after each repetition of the verse. In this new version, a participant may need all three repetitions to get in one independent clap. That's okay. The staff can encourage the action during all three repetitions, perhaps starting with hand-over-hand assistance and then shifting to verbal prompting only.

A NEW HAPPY AND YOU KNOW IT: FLOOR VERSION

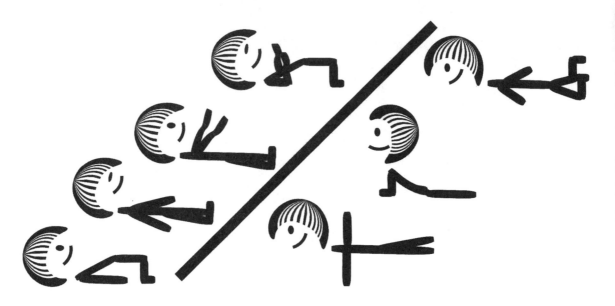

Objective

Perform new actions to familiar tunes.

Play

Play is the same as the chair version but with participants lying on the floor. Use an instrumental version of the song "If You're Happy and You Know It," or sing it without music. Each player takes a turn making up an action to one of the verses of the song. Everyone does the action.

Options

- Try it lying on the belly as well as the back.
- See the options in the chair version.

STREAMER TAG

Objective

Freeze as many players as possible in a predetermined time.

Play

One player is chosen to be the tagger and carries a paper or cloth streamer. On your signal, all the other players move in any way that they can while the tagger tries to touch them with the streamer. When touched by the streamer, the player tagged stops moving. At the end of the playing time, count those who were tagged and choose a new participant to be the tagger.

Options

- Place participants close enough for the streamer to reach. It is more important to work toward the tagger increasing his range of motion and direction of his actions than to have players placed to avoid the streamer.

- Adjust distances individually for each player who takes a turn being the tagger.

- If a participant cannot move the streamer independently, provide assistance. As always, when providing assistance, the helper must stay in constant communication with the player he is assisting. ("I will help you try to tag Mary. We need to lift your arm and swing the ribbon to the right. Here we go.") Never just move a player; always explain what is to be done and how you are going to help. Allow each participant who requires assistance the time to first try on his own.

THROW FOR DISTANCE

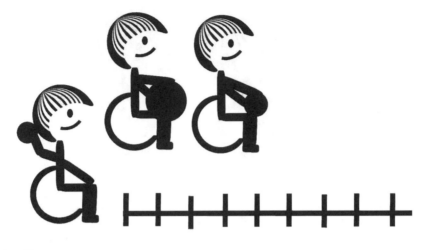

Objective

Throw, push, fling, or otherwise move a ball as far as possible.

Play

Draw a line on the floor with cross marks to indicate distance. Each player takes three turns throwing a ball, in the direction of the floor marks, as far as she can. Players can throw in whatever way that is most appropriate; the distance of each throw is recorded. The best of the three trials is used as the participant's score. Play two or more rounds with each player trying to beat her previous score. Keep a written chart or record on the wall if desired.

Options

- The size and shape of the ball should be individual to the player.
- Allow those with limited grasping or throwing ability to push a ball from the lap. Count the distance the ball rolls since that is determined by the force the player imparts to her push.
- Use this as a stand-alone activity or as an event in a larger activity such as a track and field event or Olympics.
- Repetition of the rounds can be done on the same day or on another day.

ALL OR NOTHING

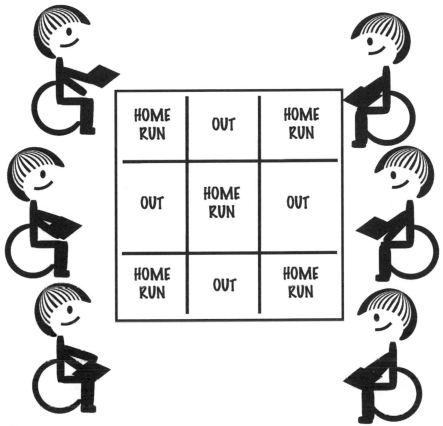

Objective

Score the most runs in the play period by tossing, throwing, or pushing beanbags or other objects onto the game mat.

Play

Create a floor game mat by drawing a tic-tac-toe style graphic on a poster board (see the illustration). In each of the resulting squares, alternate the words *home run* and *out*. Choose two teams. Members take turns tossing the beanbag to the game mat. A team scores a run if the beanbag or other object lands on a home run square and an out if it lands on an out square. Beanbags landing on the line are considered strikes; three strikes equal an out. Each team continues play until three outs are accumulated. The other team then takes their turn.

Options

- Position chairs close enough to accommodate the individual players.
- Have players participate as individuals rather than as part of a team.
- A semi-inflated ball can be used for pushing. It will drop to the game mat but not roll off.
- A game mat can be made from poster board or taped onto the floor.

Throw out the rules and make your own!

AEROBIC WORKOUT

Objective

Move continuously through one music selection.

Play

This activity is similar to an aerobics class. Play lively music with a defined beat or a song that is familiar to the players. As the music plays, call out and demonstrate different actions. Participants should follow the actions called for in the workout as best they can for the entire music piece.

Options

- Remind participants that the object is to keep moving, even if they have to substitute, modify, or continue with a movement they can do.
- Allow movements that are different from those called if a player cannot perform the indicated one. Any leg, arm, head, or body movement is okay.
- Use verbal prompting to keep everyone moving and motivated.

Warm-Up

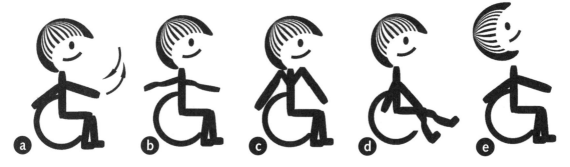

a) Inhale while raising the arms, exhale while lowering the arms.
b) Shake and wiggle arms to loosen them up.
c) Shrug the shoulders to loosen them up.
d) Shake and wiggle the legs to loosen them up.
e) Nod the head up and down and side to side.

Workout

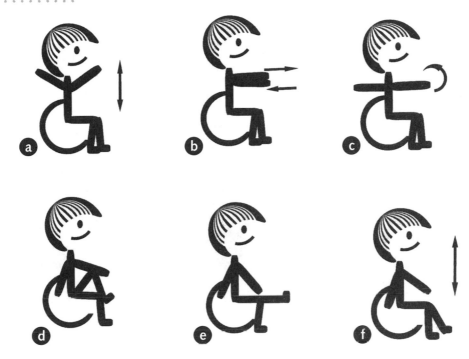

a) Lift and lower arms in **sets** of six or eight.
b) Push forward and pull back arms in sets of six or eight.
c) Perform arm circles with left arm, right arm, and then both arms together in sets of six or eight.
d) Perform alternating knee lifts in sets of six or eight.
e) Perform alternating leg lifts in sets of six or eight.
f) Alternate between lifting the right arm up and back down, lifting the left arm up and back down, lifting the right leg up and back down, and lifting the left leg up and back down.

Cool-Down

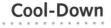

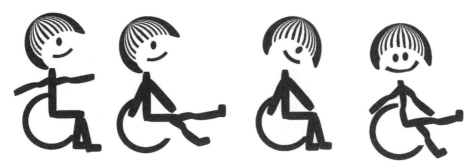

Shake out the arms, legs, head, and whole body for a count of eight.

LINE KICK

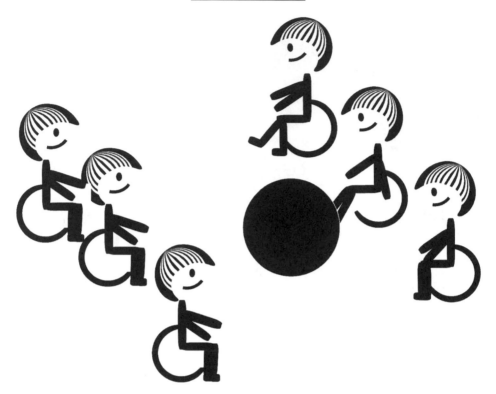

Objective

Move the ball between the two lines without it getting away.

Play

Arrange the players in two teams, chairs lined up facing one another. On your signal, a player kicks the ball toward the other line. Players on the other side return it. Play continues until the ball moves out from between the two lines. If the ball gets stuck between the two lines, a player can wheel forward to kick the ball and get it moving again. Alternatively, a staff member can give the ball a push to get it back to one of the lines.

Options

- Use a ball large enough for easy kicking.
- The two lines of chairs should be placed close enough to each other for successful play. In some cases the lines of the chairs may have to be only a short distance apart, so even a very small kick will send the ball to the other side.
- If players want to keep score, participants can score one point for every five kicks (negotiable), and the ball scores one point every time it moves out of reach.

CIRCLE KICK

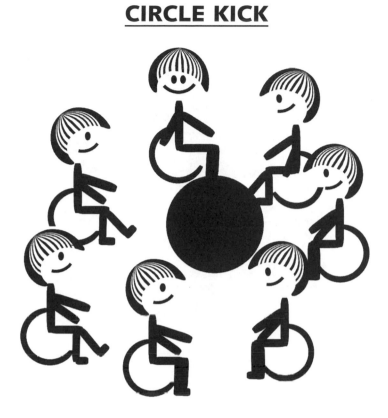

Objective

Keep the ball moving in the circle for a predetermined number of kicks.

Play

On your signal, players kick the ball around the circle trying for the targeted number of kicks before the ball escapes from the circle or comes to a stop outside of any player's reach. If the group makes the targeted number, they win the round. If not, the ball wins the round. Alternatively, count the number of successful kicks before the ball stops and try to beat that number in each of the following rounds.

Options

- Make the circle small enough to facilitate successful kicking.
- Use a ball size appropriate to the size of the circle and the ability of the players.
- Consider removing the footplates on the wheelchair so a player's legs can hang free, facilitating kicking.

TAKE A HIKE

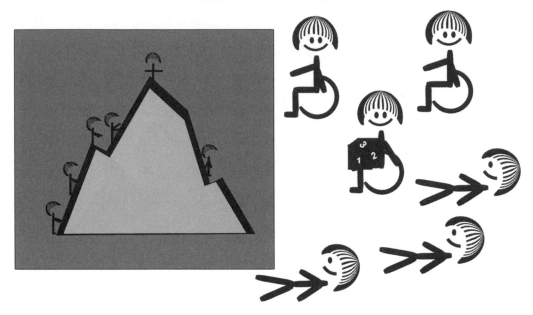

Objective

Move your game piece up and over the mountain by performing various activities.

Play

This is like a board game, with the playing board mounted on the wall for better visibility. Tape together several pieces of poster board to make a large game board and use a box to make the activity cube. Write instructions for each activity available on the activity cube and post them on the wall next to the game board. Each participant rolls the activity cube and attempts the indicated activity. If she is successful, her game piece moves one step up the mountain. If not, her game piece remains where it is on the game board. The cube is passed to the next player who takes her turn in the same way. The first player to go up, over, and down the mountain is the winner.

Options

- Activities should be a mix of easy and challenging.
- Place the game board on the wall where all participants can see it.
- If the group prefers, everyone can play until all have completed the game.
- This is a wonderful inclusion activity. It can be played in wheelchairs, on the floor, by those with limiting conditions, and by those without, all at once! The key is to make the activities fit the group. If various skill levels and abilities are present, use two or more activity cubes, each with appropriate tasks for the participants using them. Or choose activities for the cube that can be done in some way by each player.

   For example, a participant without limiting conditions could attempt to jog in place for one minute. A participant in a wheelchair might do the same activity by lifting and lowering the knees. A player on the floor might stomp her feet or simply have to move her legs to complete the activity.

- Plan a wall chart for activities that correspond to the numbers on the activity cube. Activities for use with the activity cube could include the following:
  - Do five breaths with very loud exhalations.
  - Bring your knee toward your chest three times.
  - Turn your head side to side five times.
  - Wiggle your fingers while someone counts to five.
  - Turn in a circle three times. If on the floor, roll back to front and front to back.
  - Bend forward and back four times. If on the floor, lift and lower your head and shoulders.
  - Clap your hands with your arms overhead three times.
  - Stretch your whole body. Hold the stretch for five seconds and then relax. Repeat.
  - Make circles with your arms five times in each direction.
  - Lift and lower your legs, one at a time, five times each leg.
  - Open and close your mouth five times.
  - Bend side to side very slowly, two times on each side.

OLYMPICS

Objective

As a team, complete each of the activities in an Olympic event.

Play

Choose teams and let the teams choose the country they want to represent. Make gold, silver, bronze, and Olympic participant medals out of poster board and ribbon, or purchase plastic medals in the party supply area of stores.

Each event is a team event. Scores are cumulative: Each player's score is added to the scores of the other team members. The team with the highest score for each event gets the gold. Follow up with silver, bronze, and Olympic participant medals. Hold Olympic events over several days or when the actual Olympics are held.

Options

- The events suggested are ideas only. Take any Olympic event and modify it to meet the abilities of the participants.
- Make up your own events based on the capabilities of the group.
- Within each event, make accommodations for the individual.
- Olympics can be organized as an inclusive activity. Since all events are scored as teams rather than as individuals, players of all abilities can be mixed on teams. Events should be planned to accommodate players with and without disabilities. For example, here's a 50-yard dash:
    - Players capable of running participate in an actual 50-yard dash, and their times are recorded.
    - Players in wheelchairs who can wheel themselves participate in a 10-yard dash, and their times are recorded.
    - Players who cannot propel their chairs move their legs continuously for as long as they can, and the time is recorded.
    - Add all the times of a team together to make the team score. Best score gets the gold!

Event Ideas

- One-minute dash: Each team member, in turn, moves his legs continuously for as long as he can. Record the number of seconds the player keeps moving. The times of each person on the team are added together to make the team total for the event.
- Throw or push for distance: Each player on a team pushes or throws a ball. The distance traveled is added to that of the other team members to make a team score.

- Heads-up event: Each player on a team lifts and lowers her head as many times as she can in five seconds. The number of head lifts is counted. Scores from each team member are added together to make the final team score.
- Punchball event: Each player hits the punchball repeatedly until he misses. The number of hits per individual before a miss are added together to make the team score.
- Ball drop event: Each team member must pick up and drop a sponge or squishy ball (or any appropriate ball) as many times in ten seconds as he can. The number of repetitions for each player are added together to make a team score.

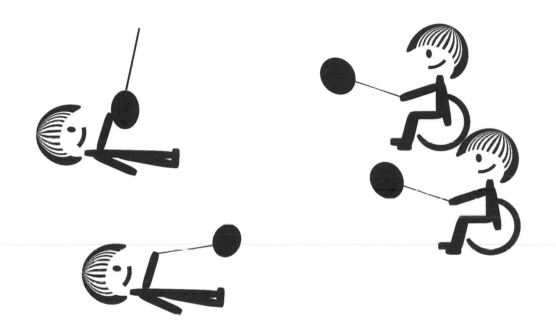

The Last Word

It is up to you to find ways to encourage independent movement and participation in physical activities when players have limiting conditions. Providing high-quality activities for those with disabilities requires dedication and creativity. There is no shortcut. Always start with what is and move toward what may be possible. Have confidence in yourself and those who participate in the activities you create.

Expect success!

About the Author

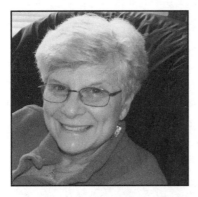

E. Ann Davis, MS, is owner of WiseSoma Health and Fitness and The Yoga Nook in Glens Falls, New York. WiseSoma Health and Fitness provides physical activity and yoga programs to children and adults of all abilities.

Davis has over 30 years of experience in the fields of physical education, recreation, therapeutic recreation, and adapted physical education working with individuals throughout the life span. As an adapted physical education teacher and a therapeutic recreation specialist, Davis has extensive experience in developing and implementing safe, successful, and creative physical activity programs for those with special needs, from infants to the elderly.

Since 1975 Davis has been sharing her experience and knowledge as a practitioner presenting programs, lectures, and workshops in the areas of elementary physical education, adapted physical education, and preschool physical education. Davis also conducts workshops on yoga for adults and children with special needs. She is a certified yoga teacher and a licensed practitioner of Yoga for the Special Child™, the Sonia Sumar method.

Davis resides in Queensbury, New York. She can be reached by email at wisesoma@yahoo.com.

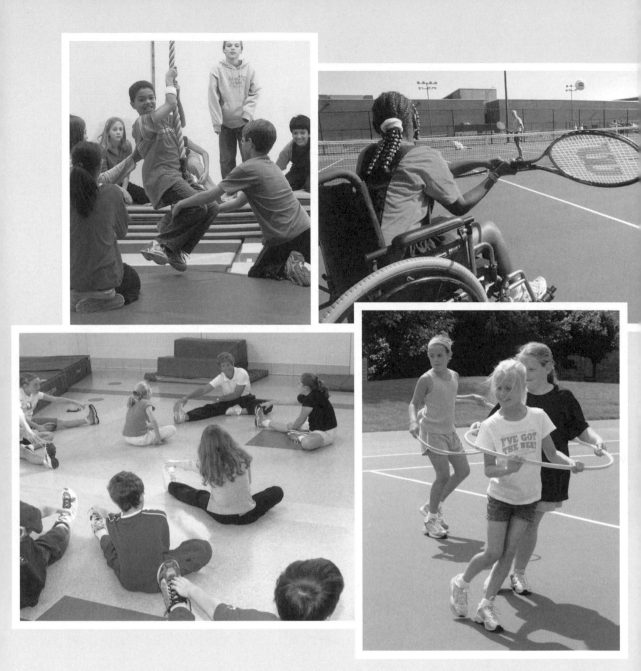

You'll find other outstanding adapted physical activity resources at
www.HumanKinetics.com